Better Buildings for Better Services:
Innovative Developments in
Primary Care

National Primary Care Research and
Development Centre Series

Better Buildings for Better Services: Innovative Developments in Primary Care

National Primary Care Research and Development Centre Series

Jackie Bailey
Caroline Glendinning
Helen Gould

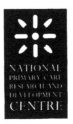

RADCLIFFE MEDICAL PRESS

Radcliffe Medical Press Ltd
18 Marcham Road, Abingdon, Oxon OX14 1AA, UK

British Library Cataloguing in Publication Data

A catalogue record for this book is available from the British Library.

ISBN 1 85775 287 2

Library of Congress Cataloging-in-Publication Data is available.

Typeset by Advance Typesetting Ltd, Oxon

The National Primary Care Research and Development Centre is a Department of Health-funded initiative, based at the University of Manchester. The NPCRDC is a multi-disciplinary centre which aims to promote high-quality and cost-effective primary care by delivering high-quality research, disseminating research findings and promoting service development based upon sound evidence. The Centre has staff based at three collaborating sites: The National Centre at the University of Manchester, The Public Health Research and Resource Centre at the University of Salford and the Centre for Health Economics at the University of York.

For further information about the Centre or a copy of our research prospectus please contact

Maria Cairney
Communications Officer, NPCRDC
The University of Manchester
5th Floor, Williamson Building
Oxford Road
Manchester M13 9PL

Tel: 0161 275 7633/7601

Contents

About the authors

Jackie Bailey is Research Fellow at the National Primary Care Research and Development Centre, University of Manchester.

Caroline Glendinning is Senior Research Fellow at the National Primary Care Research and Development Centre, University of Manchester.

Helen Gould is Research Associate at the National Primary Care Research and Development Centre, University of Manchester.

Acknowledgements

We are particularly grateful to the project leaders and other staff involved in the innovative developments described in this book. They willingly gave up their time to talk to us and provide detailed information about the developments with which they were involved. We hope that the short summaries contained in this book do justice to their achievements.

Within the NPCRDC, Yvonne Burkey helped with the initial identification of study sites. Many thanks are due to Catherine Bewley who stepped in at short notice to help with the fieldwork and who provided clear and succinct summaries of the case studies. Margarita Cook provided administrative support and Maria Cairney, Tom Butler and Lisa Tilsley gave advice and administrative support with dissemination. Gillian Nineham helped to steer this book through the Radcliffe Medical Press publication process.

The research on which this book is based was commissioned by NHS Estates. However, the findings and conclusions of the study are the sole responsibility of the authors.

Caroline Glendinning
July 1997

Abbreviations

CAB	Citizens Advice Bureau
CHC	Community Health Council
CPN	Community Psychiatric Nurse
DBFO	Design, Build, Finance, Operate
EU	European Union
FHSA	Family Health Services Authority
GMS	General Medical Services
GP	General Practitioner
HCHS	Hospital and Community Health Services
LIZ	London Initiative Zone
LMC	Local Medical Committee
PFI	Private Finance Initiative
RDA	Rural Development Area
SFA	Statement of Fees and Allowances
SRB	Single Regeneration Budget (incorporating City Challenge)
VFM	Value for Money

1

Primary care –
policy and premises

INTRODUCTION

Over the past few years, primary health services have moved firmly into the centre of the NHS policy agenda. During 1996, a number of White Papers were introduced to support the development of a 'primary care-led NHS'.[1,2,3] The *NHS (Primary Care) Act 1997* which followed will enable selected pilot sites to experiment with new arrangements for providing primary care services. Pilot sites might be led by GPs, community trusts or partnerships of different providers. They are likely to develop new approaches to the commissioning and provision of primary care, e.g. the employment of salaried doctors. The impact on the future shape of primary and community health services is potentially profound.

New developments in primary health services will place new demands on premises: to accommodate professionals who have previously worked in separate locations; to house equipment and services transferred from hospital to community settings; and to provide accommodation for the local voluntary and community groups whose involvement is a key feature of many new primary health service developments. Sometimes new buildings will be needed; on other occasions the renovation or extension of existing premises will be required. Within overall public expenditure constraints, capital funding for such developments may be difficult to obtain. Furthermore, conventional sources of capital may simply not be appropriate for complex, multi-service developments.

A number of pioneer developments in primary health services have already tackled this challenge. Ten such developments form the focus of this book. They illustrate the twin challenges of developing new patterns of primary and community-based health services and funding and designing appropriate buildings in which these services can be housed. The ten initiatives represent a range of different service development objectives and finance procurement strategies that include developments led by GP practices, health authorities, acute and community NHS trusts. They draw on private finance packages secured by GP practices; partnerships with private development companies; finance raised from regional and district health authorities; capital raised in partnership with local authorities from regeneration programmes such as City Challenge, Single Regeneration Budget and the Rural Development Commission; and capital grants from charitable foundations. In some cases these initiatives have had to adapt the conventional routes for securing the capital and revenue funding needed to pay for new primary care premises; other traditional routes may become less available as structural changes in the NHS are implemented. They illustrate an expanding range of options for financing premises for primary care.

The innovative projects described in this book are not intended to be definitive models or 'blueprints'. Decisions about service configurations and funding strategies will always need to be made in the light of local circumstances, constraints and opportunities. Instead, these innovative projects illustrate the wide range of solutions that can be found to the common problems of limited local services and restricted or inadequate premises from which to expand and improve those services. They provide a glimpse into the future of primary and community health services – an illustration of how services and premises could develop into the next millennium. Although they may appear to be at the 'leading edge' of primary care development, they illustrate the range of opportunities that are likely to be available in the future.

GPs will remain at the heart of primary care services and traditional sources of funding to support GPs in owning or renting their premises will remain. However, the pilot sites promised by the 1997 Act will open up new avenues and opportunities. Many of these opportunities will require close collaboration between GPs, health authorities and trusts, local authorities, private sector finance, property design and development companies, universities and charitable organizations. Increasingly, there will be pressures to involve local communities as well. Some of these alliances will, in the first instance, be forged by the desire to increase the accessibility of services and improve collaboration across organizational and professional boundaries; others will be driven initially by the need to put together complex packages of capital funding from a number of different sources.

However, one of the key lessons from the ten innovative developments described in this book is that the processes of service development and premises development are interactive. New service objectives will shape building specifications and capital funding options; conversely, the need to secure capital and revenue income is likely to influence the services which are based in new developments. As the opportunities introduced by the 1997 Act take effect, the complex processes involved in developing primary and community health services will become increasingly apparent, especially if such developments also aim to achieve better co-operation across service boundaries and closer partnerships with local communities.

THE NEED TO DEVELOP AND IMPROVE
PRIMARY CARE PREMISES

Primary Care: Delivering the Future acknowledged that residual problems remain with a small number of premises which are still not 'adequate for the provision of personal, hygienic care'.[3] However, far more extensive problems arise from the restrictions that many existing GP practice and health centre premises impose on the further expansion and diversification of primary and community-based health services.

Primary care is no longer restricted just to GP, dental, optician and community pharmacy services or even those provided by an expanded practice-based team. Rather, it encompasses a broad network of community health services provided in or near to patients' homes, which together enables 90% of all health care in the UK to be managed outside hospitals. As NHS policies and technological developments continue to encourage services to be moved from distant hospitals to community settings, primary care will also increasingly include more specialized services (e.g. diagnostic services, rehabilitation services, or treatment for people with moderate or severe mental health problems), as well as generalist community-based services such as district nursing and health visiting. In some of the innovative developments described in this book, the definition of primary care is being extended yet further, in acknowledgement of the important role that local communities can play in improving the physical and mental well-being of their residents.[4,5]

The following section summarizes a number of longer-term changes and pressures, which arguably have transformed the nature and scope of primary health services over recent years. It is important that the premises within which primary care services are provided can be adapted and developed to accommodate the expanded range of services that are already found within primary and community health settings and that are likely to become even more common in future.

Changes in the scope of primary health services

The diversity of services provided within primary care has expanded very considerably since the beginning of the 1990s. The revised GP contract in 1990 and the introduction of GP fundholding in 1991 have together brought about major changes to the scope of general medical services provided by GPs. Practice nurses, nurse practitioners with more extensive treatment and prescribing responsibilities, other specialist nurses and paramedical staff are now often members of the primary health care team. Counselling, physiotherapy and specialist outpatient clinics are also now frequently based in GP premises.

The introduction of additional payments to GPs for providing specific services has also resulted in an increase in activities such as child health surveillance, health promotion, chronic disease management and minor surgical procedures. GP fundholding has also provided a major impetus to this expansion and diversification, as the various types of budget-holding have offered some financial flexibility and, therefore, increased opportunities for innovation and change in the provider roles of primary care as well as in the purchasing of secondary services.[6] This expansion of primary care services has been accompanied by the need to invest in service management; practice managers are now the norm rather than the exception.[7]

These developments in primary care services have had major implications for primary care premises. More clinical accommodation is needed; premises also need to be larger than the traditional surgery in order to accommodate new equipment. Multi-functional accommodation will also commonly be required, for services that are provided on a sessional basis.

Information technology in primary care has developed rapidly. Computerized patient record systems are becoming the norm; computer terminals and fax machines need to be accommodated on GPs' desks alongside the traditional stethoscope and prescription pad. Some GP practices are now experimenting with telemedicine links with hospital-based clinicians who can offer specialist diagnoses and advice about treatment.[8] Although still at an early experimental stage, such links will place further pressures on available accommodation if they become more widespread.

Changes in the primary care workforce

A further pressure for change is the changing nature of the GP and primary care workforce itself. As indicated above, there has been a dramatic increase in the numbers and range of staff now working within primary health care teams. The entry of significant numbers of women into general practice has created additional pressures for alternatives to the traditional long-term investment in practice premises that has hither to accompanied GP principal status.[9] Increased demands for part-time employment opportunities, more flexible career paths and the introduction of salaried options for GPs following the 1997 legislation all call for the development of additional capital investment options and property ownership arrangements in primary care.

The strategic shift from secondary to primary care

Since the early 1990s, NHS policies have encouraged the movement of diagnostic and treatment-related services from hospitals to community and primary care settings. Both the payment system introduced by the 1990 GP contract and the expansion of GP fundholding have facilitated these developments. More extensive and invasive procedures such as endoscopy can now be provided within primary care, albeit within a clear regulatory framework.[10] GPs seeking financial remuneration for such work are required to enter into special 'add-on' contracts with their health authority for this work, which falls outside the scope of general medical services.

The provision of such services outside traditional hospital settings (particularly where general anaesthesia is involved) clearly requires specialized extra accommodation in which to house equipment, treatment and recovery rooms.

Intermediate care

The boundaries between primary and secondary health services are shifting in other respects with the development of schemes to support seriously ill people in the community, facilitate early hospital discharge or prevent 'inappropriate' hospital admission.[11,12] Schemes of this type typically bring intensive nursing, convalescence and rehabilitation services, such as physiotherapy and occupational therapy, within the scope of primary care services. GPs may retain responsibility for managing patients and making decisions about inpatient admissions (e.g. for assessment or respite care), and for providing domiciliary services on discharge. Some intermediate care schemes involve the (re)development of small local hospitals to provide a flexible mixture of inpatient nursing beds and local outpatient treatment and therapy services.[13] It is likely that as increasing numbers of very frail older people with complex health problems are supported in the community, the need for flexible, intensive nursing facilities managed within primary care will increase.

Changes in medical training

A further consequence of the shift from secondary to primary care is the impact on professional training, both before and after initial qualification. Both doctors and nurses now need to receive an increased proportion of their initial training in community settings.[14] The development of practice-based continuing medical education may place further pressure on accommodation within primary care premises in future.

Changes in the organization of out-of-hours services

A continuing issue of contention within primary care is the contractual obligation on GPs to provide 24-hour emergency medical care. The 1995 agreement between the Department of Health and the British Medical Association included an allocation of £90 million over two years, much of which has been used to establish co-operatives between groups of GPs and practices, out-of-hours emergency centres and other alternatives to the traditional night-time home visit. Patients are encouraged to visit such centres wherever possible, particularly during the evening and at weekends, and many co-operatives provide telephone advice services. Out-of-hours centres can provide a base for other services such as district nurses, mobile wardens and social work teams who are on duty outside office hours.

Premises for out-of-hours services require facilities for carrying out treatments and domestic facilities for staff on duty during the evening and night. Out-of-hours premises also require comprehensive security systems, particularly in the urban areas where they are most likely to be found.

Widening definitions of health – the inter-agency agenda

Finally, there has been a growing recognition that health status is not determined solely by the primary and other health care services available to the local population, but by a range of other social, environmental and economic factors as well. Some innovative primary care developments are therefore seeking to address these factors in order to maximize physical and mental well-being. Leisure facilities, 'prescriptions' for exercise, and alternative therapies such as acupuncture and aromatherapy are increasingly to be found in mainstream primary care premises, alongside more conventional treatment facilities.

There is a further dimension to this wider health agenda – the growing recognition that inter-agency collaboration can reduce fragmentation between services and maximize health gain. In many instances this does not simply involve better communication or closer working between different professional groups, statutory and voluntary organizations; it means increasing the accessibility of these services to patients as well. For example, primary health care teams concerned about levels of material deprivation might seek to increase take-up of social security benefits by offering welfare rights and money advice sessions; others concerned about the poor health of ethnic minority patients might wish to introduce an interpreting and advocacy service. Particular problems at the interfaces between health and social care services are creating pressures for closer collaboration with social services departments, in order to improve the co-ordination of community care and mental health services. Again, all these service developments place pressure on the accommodation available within traditional GP surgery and health centre premises.

ABOUT THIS BOOK

Many existing primary care premises may be too small or otherwise inappropriate to accommodate an expanded range of primary and community health services. A series of regulatory and other changes have been proposed that will make it easier for GPs and health authorities to address the specific needs of local communities.[3] Current funding options and the proposed changes are described in Chapter 2.

The main focus of this book is a description of ten innovative capital and service developments in primary health care. These initiatives, summarized in Chapter 3, illustrate a wide range of different solutions to the common problems of limited local services and restricted premises from which to expand and improve those services. In each development, information was obtained through interviews carried out with the lead players; these usually included health authority officers as well as general practice and/or trust staff. The interviews were supplemented where possible with documentary evidence, such as the project's business case.

Chapter 4 draws together the experiences of these new capital developments in primary care. It discusses the benefits and drawbacks of different capital procurement options and the lessons of good project management, service development and collaborative working that can be learnt from these innovations.

REFERENCES

1   Department of Health (1996) *Primary Care: The Future*. Department of Health, London.

2   Department of Health (1996) *Primary Care: The Future – Choice and Opportunity*. Department of Health, London.

3   Department of Health (1996) *Primary Care: Delivering the Future*. Department of Health, London.

4   Gillam S, Plamping D, McClenahan J and Harries J (1994) *Community-oriented Primary Care*. King's Fund, London.

5   Harrison L and Neve F (1996) *A Review of Innovations in Primary Care*. The Policy Press, Bristol.

6   Glennerster H, Matsaganis M and Owens P (1994) *Implementing GP Fundholding*. Open University Press, Buckingham.

7   Huntington J (1995) *Managing the Practice: whose business?* Radcliffe Medical Press, Oxford.

8   Harrison R, Clayton W and Wallace P (1996) Can telemedicine be used to improve communication between primary and secondary care? *BMJ*. **313**: 1377–81.

9   Allen I (1992) *Part-time Working in General Practice*. Policy Studies Institute, London.

10 NHSE (1996) *A National Framework for the Provision of Secondary Care Within General Practice, HSG(96)31*. NHS Executive, Leeds.

11 Pederson LL and Leese B (1997) What will a primary care-led NHS mean for GP workload? The problem of the lack of an evidence base. *BMJ*. **314**: 1337–41.

12 Gordon P and Hadley J (eds) (1996) *Extending Primary Care: polyclinics, resource centres, hospitals-at-home*. Radcliffe Medical Press, Oxford.

13 Newman P and Crown J (1996) *Intermediate Care: a literature review*. In: *Intermediate Care Resource Pack*. NHSE, Anglia and Oxford Region.

14 GMC (1993) *Tomorrow's Doctors: recommendations on undergraduate medical education*. General Medical Council, London.

2

Funding arrangements for primary care capital developments

Many GP practice premises and health centres are neither suitable nor large enough to meet the changes and challenges outlined in Chapter 1. Buildings within which health services are accommodated must be adaptable, flexible and responsive to changing patterns of use. There are major constraints on premises development, including the availability of suitable land or property, and urban areas have particular problems in lack of space for expansion. Perhaps the largest constraint, however, is obtaining the necessary capital funding to build new premises or convert/refurbish existing properties.

The White Paper, *Primary Care: Delivering the Future*, outlines a range of changes that are intended to increase funding flexibilities within continuing overall restrictions on public sector capital expenditure.[1] These changes are aimed at increasing the range of flexibilities available to health authorities to address specific local needs and at facilitating the development of higher quality and larger, more flexible, primary care premises. The following sections outline the available current funding options for premises development and the changes proposed by the White Paper (sections in italics). No firm timetable has been given for most of these changes and their implementation may be affected by the change of government in May 1997.

COST RENT SCHEME

The cost rent scheme is administered by health authorities to reimburse GPs who wish to improve surgery premises, either by building new premises, acquiring premises for substantial modification or substantially modifying existing premises, for the provision of General Medical Services.[2] This scheme enables GPs to be reimbursed the costs of funding the development subject to a prescribed interest rate on the cost and up to limits set out in the Statement of Fees and Allowances (SFA). These limits depend on the size of the practice and include maximum floor areas and costs. Additional spaces can be allocated and cost allowances claimed for attached nursing staff, common room, trainee room, assessment room and a dispensary. The limits set out in the SFA date from the 1970s and are inadequate for modern-day primary care, e.g. room sizes are not sufficient.[3] If the planned accommodation is built larger than outlined in the SFA, then the cost of any additional space will not be reimbursed under the scheme. Any resulting shortfall from higher building costs or larger room sizes have to be met from the GPs own resources. Cost rent continues to be reimbursed to GPs until notional rent is deemed to be more beneficial by the GPs (see below). Total cost rent expenditure is cash-limited at the health authority level. With few practices converting to notional rent in the recent past due to the decline of property values, little funding is available for new projects. However, with the ongoing recovery of the housing market this may be a temporary situation.

The White Paper proposes the introduction of new cost rent schedules to allow funding for a larger size and wider range of facilities within premises.

NOTIONAL RENT REIMBURSEMENT

Notional rent is reimbursed to all GPs not receiving cost rent, who own and finance their surgery premises. The amount of notional rent is based on the District Valuer's assessment of the current market rent that may be expected to be paid for the premises and is reviewed every three years. Notional rent is not cash-limited and there are therefore incentives for health authorities to move as many GPs as possible from cost rent to notional rent (or actual rent schemes). However, the move from cost rent to notional rent is irrevocable and problems have arisen when practices have found that the notional rent falls below the original cost rent, sometimes resulting in negative equity problems.

ACTUAL RENT REIMBURSEMENT

Payments to reimburse GPs who rent their premises will be the lease rent or current market rent as assessed by the District Valuer, whichever is the less. Actual rent reimbursement is not cash-limited. From April 1997, GPs who have leases or licences in health centres became eligible for reimbursement for rent and rates by health authorities up to the limit of the current market rent set by the District Valuer.

Guidance has recently been sent out by NHS Estates outlining the requirement to establish a real cash rental flow between GPs and NHS trusts (as the owners of the health centres).[4] This also includes the ability of GPs to apply to health authorities for improvement grants.

An NHS Executive/Valuation Office survey in 1995/96 shows that 63% of premises are owned by GPs and reimbursed by either cost rent (30%) or notional rent (33%); 16% are owned by trusts or health authorities (the latter acting on behalf of the Secretary of

State) and are now to be reimbursed by actual rent; and 21% are owned by private landlords and reimbursed by actual rent.[5] Recent years have witnessed a marked decline in property and rental values – this has implications for cost and notional rent schemes and may have implications for future private sector funding as these values recover.

IMPROVEMENT GRANTS

These grants from health authorities can be used to expand and improve surgery accommodation but cannot be used to build new premises or purchase land. They are cash-limited and GPs may obtain one to two-thirds of the cost of the improvements (or up to 90% within the London Initiative Zone until the end of March 1999).

FUNDHOLDER SAVINGS

Many GP fundholders have used savings to make improvements to their surgeries to provide a more comprehensive range of services to their patients, e.g. to build extra treatment rooms for community nurses or visiting consultants.[6] To date savings cannot be used to purchase land or property.[7] The fundholder must secure agreement from the health authority for the proposed use of savings and the changes should provide 'value for money' (VFM) to the NHS and the taxpayer. The use of fundholder savings is a contentious issue as fundholders may be able to acquire increased equity on retirement.[3]

The White Paper suggests that new arrangements governing fundholder savings might permit the purchase of land or new buildings, subject to safeguards regarding VFM and benefits for patients.

NHS TRUSTS

Trusts can borrow funding for premises subject to their agreed external finance limit (EFL). Other funding sources for trusts may result from the trusts' estates strategies and could include property and land sales. Trust capital and property assets are now valued and depreciated in their balance sheets and trusts are required to meet an appropriate capital charge on the value of assets employed. As mentioned above, trusts can bid for treasury capital through regional offices by preparing full business cases.

NHS EXECUTIVE REGIONAL OFFICES AND HEALTH AUTHORITIES

In 1996, NHS Executive regional offices replaced regional health authorities and health authorities replaced district health authorities and family health services authorities. Funding from regional offices and health authorities may often be linked to hospital closures or other rationalization or disinvestment in secondary care. NHS trusts may apply for capital against their EFL from regional offices. Some regional offices and health authorities have also offered pump priming monies to enable schemes to move forward, although this may not always be available.[5]

Proposals in the White Paper will enable health authorities to use loans and grants to help GPs move out of sub-standard premises. These may enable GPs on long-term leases to buy out the leases if they agree to invest in improved premises; and may encourage single-handed GPs to move to shared premises.

London Initiative Zone (LIZ)

In London, capital funds (known as Tomlinson or LIZ monies) were earmarked for primary care development to support a proposed reduction in hospital services. LIZ covers four million people and consists of those areas where health care needs are high and primary care provision is weak. Over 60% of LIZ monies have gone into expanding the range and quality of primary care premises.[8] LIZ allows greater flexibility for health authorities to hold land and allows for 90% improvement grants, along with the usual capital resource availability. Initially the initiative was managed by the London Implementation Group, which was superseded by the Primary Care Support Force; this is now an NHS Executive regional office function. However, this extra funding is time-limited and all money is accounted for until the end of March 1999.

Private finance

GPs and private funding arrangements

GPs have always been able to access private finance in approximately the same way as any small business and with little bureaucracy and regulation. GP-led schemes with the private sector have to date been easier to progress than those led by trusts since there is generally no need to produce business cases or to satisfy various conditions (e.g. delivering VFM). GPs can secure favourable loans from banks and other lending institutions that frequently offer attractive rates. However, there are disincentives for GPs taking on loans, including the high initial costs, the risk of negative equity, reduced mobility and reduced personal financial freedom.

Private Finance Initiative (PFI)

PFI allows private sector contractors to design, build, finance and operate (DBFO) premises. PFI is intended to draw additional capital investment and private sector construction, financial planning skills and facilities management into the public sector and it has been promoted as the means of maintaining overall levels of capital investment in the NHS and of introducing innovative solutions to the issue of premises.[9] However, so far the DBFO model developed within the hospital context has rarely been used in primary settings, because the size of primary care premises does not make facilities and building management a financially attractive proposition to private firms. Major conditions for approving PFI schemes are that they should demonstrate an appropriate allocation of risk to the private sector and that they should provide VFM. Private developers may be interested in funding *new building construction*, retaining the freehold and granting leases to health care providers; they may wish to invest in *existing buildings* that they then upgrade and improve, offering either sale or leaseback to GPs; or they may invest in *mixed use* projects, including commercial space for shops or housing.

However, PFI is alleged to have problems.[10] It potentially locks NHS organizations into long-term revenue-based contracts that may reduce responsiveness to changing needs; its associated rules and bureaucracy are complex (although these do not currently apply to GP premises); and rapid timetables result in less time for user consultation. Under current financial rules, NHS buildings have a lifespan of up to 60 years, whereas PFI developers want to secure a return on their investment over 25–30 years.[11] This can result in higher charges to the NHS and parties are tied in for a lengthy period, at the end of which they may have to renew the lease on increasingly uncompetitive market terms. Primary care developments may be too small to interest private developers and therefore health authorities, GPs and trusts may need to consider co-locating surgeries together into 'super surgeries', if appropriate to local circumstances. There may be less scope for full DBFO schemes as primary care facilities management may not be attractive to the private sector. However, a private developer can often offer a fresh location for the services in DBFO schemes.

Some of these problems may be addressed in negotiation with the developers about the lease, market rates, capped rent reviews, break clauses and obtaining a share of profit if the building is sold, as has happened in an example of a primary care PFI in Bolton.[9]

The White Paper encourages the use of private investment for GP premises development through PFI. New guidance is currently being drawn up for GPs, the NHS generally and private developers.

The current method of premises valuation could affect future private sector funding of premises. Valuations of health properties have until now been based on the commercial value of premises if they ceased to be health services facilities, e.g. if they reverted to a shop or other commercial use. In poorer, inner city areas this has necessarily meant a low valuation, which may be too low to allow private developers a viable financial return on capital investment. Recent reports suggest that the situation has been changing, at least in London.[12] This has resulted from a slight upward turn in the property market and from developers working closely with District Valuers to justify higher valuations for health premises. There is also a move to have a separate category for health buildings and a more standardized approach by District Valuers.

OTHER SOURCES OF FUNDING

There is a range of further funding sources that may be used to bring together a 'package' of capital funding.

Single Regeneration Budget

This came into effect in April 1994 and pulls together the resources from 20 programmes, including City Challenge, Task Forces and Urban Development Corporations. A proportion of the total annual budget has been made available for new regeneration schemes (the 'challenge fund'). Funding is allocated yearly on a competitive basis to local partnerships that produce plans for regeneration of their areas. Most initiatives are led by local authorities or Training and Enterprise Councils (TECs). The emphasis of the challenge fund is on strong partnerships, involvement of communities, strong links with the private sector and evidence of need. Indicators of 'need' take into account unemployment, poverty levels and health. Those bids that succeed have an integrated strategy for a specific geographical area, incorporating a full package of housing, health and community development. Bids may complement or relate to other regional and local initiatives such as local public health strategies, e.g. drug action teams. Matched resources have to be identified, e.g. from private developers, and these resources need not necessarily be cash – they could instead be the expertise and staffing provided from, for example, the local authority.

European sources

European Union Structural Funds are aimed at redressing economic disparities within the Union in areas of industrial and agricultural decline and high deprivation. Fourteen regions of England and Wales are eligible for assistance. Bids are prepared by partnerships of local organizations. The main area of health care in which the EU is involved concerns public health – the 1995–99 programme covers several fields of activity, notably cancer, AIDS, drug addiction, nutrition, tobacco and alcohol consumption.

Rural Challenge Programme

The government's Rural Challenge Programme provides six annual prizes of £1 million to be spent over three years in priority Rural Development Areas (RDAs). The competition aims to stimulate the formation of innovative new partnerships to tackle particular economic and social problems. In each RDA, a partnership involving the Rural Development Commission, local authorities, Rural Community Councils and other key public, private and voluntary sector organizations, prepare a strategy assessing the RDA's economic and social needs and priorities.

Mental Health Challenge Fund[13]

This fund was initiated in 1996/97 for new mental health service developments where health authorities provided matched funding. Projects supported by the Fund include new crisis intervention centres and beds in special 24-hour nursed care units. The Fund will operate on the same basis in 1997/98.

Charitable trusts and foundations

Funding may be available from a wide range of charitable sources, although it is usually for relatively small amounts.

THE FUTURE FOR CAPITAL DEVELOPMENTS IN PRIMARY CARE

The traditional funding mechanisms as outlined above are likely to continue to form the basis for most capital projects in primary care, alongside the possibility of some new opportunities for partnerships with the private sector. However, innovative service developments may prompt a need for additional funding mechanisms and sources, and additional impetus for new premises developments may come from the proposals outlined in *Primary Care: Delivering the Future*.[1] These have been supported by an extra £65 million in General Medical Services cash-limited funds for 1997/98 to enable health authorities 'to develop primary care through existing mechanisms and take advantage of the additional flexibilities and initiatives in this White Paper'.[1] Future funding arrangements are likely to be obtained through public and private sector partnerships. The case studies in Chapter 3 highlight what can be achieved when innovative approaches to capital funding are applied to innovative service developments.

REFERENCES

1 Department of Health (1996) *Primary Care: Delivering the Future*. Department of Health, London.

2 Ellis N and Chisholm J (1997) *Making Sense of the Red Book* (3rd ed.). Radcliffe Medical Press, Oxford.

3 Chidgey S (1996) Primary care premises: the options now available. *Primary Care Management*. **6**: 10–12.

4 NHSE (1997) *GP Occupation of Health Centres, FHSL(97)20*. NHS Executive, Leeds.

5 Fallon P (1996) Presentation at *Designing for a Healthier Future* conference, Bristol.

6 Audit Commission (1996) *What the Doctor Ordered: a study of GP fundholders in England and Wales*. HMSO, London.

7 NHSE (1995) *GP Fundholding: use of savings, HSG(95)46*. NHS Executive, Leeds.

8   Mays N, Morley V, Boyle S, Newman P *et al.* (1997) *Evaluating Primary Care Development.* King's Fund, London.

9   Kirk S and Glendinning C (1997) Using private finance in primary care. *Primary Care Management.* In press.

10 Dawson D and Maynard A (1996) Private finance for the public good? *BMJ.* **313**: 312.

11 Dix A (1997) DoH unveils 'stopgap' NHS loans to boost PFI projects. *Health Service Journal.* **107**(5537): 8.

12 Morris N (1997) Niche opportunity. *Health Service Journal* (Special Report). **107**(5542): 9–10.

13 Developing partnerships in mental health (CM 3555). (1997) The Stationery Office, London.

3

Innovative primary care developments: case studies

Ten primary care developments were studied. They ranged from a GP practice moving to new premises funded by a private developer, to a polyclinic collaboration between two NHS trusts funded by a combination of capital grants from the NHS regional executive, the local authority and one of the trusts.

Table 3.1 shows the range of capital funding mechanisms, key players and opening dates, and Table 3.2, the actual or planned service provision for each site. Summaries of the case studies follow that describe the aims and key players, funding sources, ownership and management, service provision and key features. A list of key contacts for each of the study sites can be found in Appendix 1, followed by a detailed breakdown of the service packages and service providers in Appendix 2.

Table 3.1: Summary of case studies

Site	Description	Funding source	Cost	Key players	Opening date
Belmont Medical Centre Uxbridge, Middlesex	– Office conversion – GP premises	– Private developer	£1.25 million	– Developer – GP practice – Health authority	August 1996
Hebden Bridge Group Practice, Hebden Bridge, West Yorkshire	– Mill conversion – GP premises – Secondary health care services	– Private developer	Unknown	– Developer – GP practice – Health authority	January 1998
Hove Polyclinic Hove, East Sussex	– New building – Acute trust services – Community trust services – No GPs	– NHS trust – Regional health authority	£4.9 million	– Health authority – NHS trusts	1998
Kiveton Park Health Centre Kiveton Park South Yorkshire	– New building – GP premises – Voluntary/community agencies	– GP commercial loan – RDA grant – Health authority	£1.03 million	– GP practice – Health authority	January 1997
Neptune Health Park Tipton, West Midlands	– New building – Equal partnership approach – GP premises – Combined trust services – Voluntary/community agencies	– NHS trust – City Challenge	£3.2 million	– GP practice – Community/vol. – NHS trust – Health authority – City Challenge	June 1998
Northwich Centre for Integrated Care Northwich, Cheshire	– New build and listed building conversion – Acute trust services – Community trust services – Voluntary/community agencies	– Regional health authority	£1.2 million	– Health authority – NHS trust	July 1997

Table 3.1: *continued*

Site	Description	Funding source	Cost	Key players	Opening date
Richford Gate Primary Care Centre, Richford Gate, West London	– GP practice – Community trust services – Commercial letting units	– LIZ	£1 million	– GP practice – Health authority – NHS trust	June 1996
Shadwell Medical Centre Leeds, West Yorkshire	– Conversion of empty property – GP premises – Commercial letting units	– GP commercial loan	£299 500	– GP practice	November 1994
St Matthew's Health and Community Centre Leicester, Leicestershire	– Conversion of former residential home – GP premises – Community trust services – Voluntary/community agencies – Mental health trust services – Social services, Benefits Agency, police	– NHS trust – Regional health authority – Health authority – Charities – Local authority – City Challenge	£2.12 million	– GP practice – NHS trust – Community – Health authority – Local authority	July 1996
West End Health Resource Centre Newcastle-upon-Tyne, Tyne and Wear	– New building – GP premises – Community trust services – Fitness and leisure facilities – Voluntary/community agencies	– Regional health authority – City Challenge – University	£1.23 million	– GP practice – Regional office – Health authority – Community – NHS trust	May 1996

Table 3.2: Summary of service provision

Services	Belmont Medical Centre	Hebden Bridge GP	Hove Poly-clinic	Kiveton Park HC	Neptune Health Park	Northwich CIC	Richford Gate PCC	Shadwell Medical Centre	St Matthew's HCC	West End HRC
▲ **GP services**										
General practitioner and GMS	•	•		•	•		•	•	•	•
Out-of-hours care	•	•	•	•	•		•	•	•	
Minor surgery			•		•	•	•	•		
▲ **Community services**										
Community nursing (e.g. district nursing, health visitors)	•	•	•		•	•	•	•	•	
Community services (e.g. chiropody, health promotion)	•	•	•	•	•	•	•	•	•	•
▲ **Physiotherapy**	•	•	•	•	•		•	•		•
▲ **Mental health services** (e.g. CPN, counselling)	•		•	•	•		•	•	•	•
▲ **Social services** (e.g. care assessments)					•		•			•
▲ **Secondary care services**										
Outpatient clinics			•		•	•				
Diagnostic facilities (e.g. radiology)			•		•	•				
Day case surgery			•		•	•				
Telemedicine/remote diagnosis		•				•				
▲ **Rehabilitation services**					•	•				
▲ **Minor injuries unit**	•				•	•				•

Table 3.2: *continued*

Services	Belmont Medical Centre	Hebden Bridge GP	Hove Poly-clinic	Kiveton Park HC	Neptune Health Park	Northwich CIC	Richford Gate PCC	Shadwell Medical Centre	St Matthew's HCC	West End HRC
▲ **Information and advice services** (e.g. CAB)									•	•
▲ **Teaching facilities**					•	•	•		•	•
▲ **Community groups access**			•	•	•	•	•		•	•
▲ **Voluntary organizations**				•	•	•			•	•
▲ **Complementary therapies** (e.g. massage)					•	•	•			•
▲ **Other private practitioners**										
Dentist					•		•			
Pharmacy			•		•		•	•	•	
Optician					•		•	•		
▲ **Leisure/fitness facilities**										•

BELMONT MEDICAL CENTRE: UXBRIDGE

Development:	New GP premises
Funding:	Private developer
Capital cost:	£1 250 000
Timescale:	1994–August 1996

Profile

The investment from a private developer in this project enabled the GP practice to escape from the trap caused by high property prices and lack of cost rent funding. The practice now leases much larger premises and has taken on the responsibility for managing and maintaining the building in order to qualify for a higher reimbursement under the SFA regulations. The private developer acted as a broker between the practice and the health authority.

Aims and key players

The practice had been trying to move to larger premises for some years and was frustrated by the lack of suitable property and the potential high costs as owner-occupiers in an area with high property costs. A previous failed expansion plan had lost the practice a substantial amount of money and made it receptive to the rental option. The practice was keen to exploit some of the opportunities available to it as a community fundholder; it wanted to arrest a decline in list size and to enhance the range of services provided. At that time, the FHSA had a policy of supporting opportunistic premises developments. At the outset, the key players were the practice, the developer, Primary Health Care Centres (PHCC) and the FHSA. PHCC is a private development company specializing in health care sites. Following the merger of the

FHSA and the District Health Authority, the newly formed Hillingdon Health Authority took on a leading role. Throughout the process, PHCC worked to the practice's specification and led the negotiations about funding and lease arrangements with the health authority and District Valuer.

Funding

PHCC found a suitable site; an empty office block with adjoining car park in Uxbridge. The building was owned by an insurance company and leased to British Petroleum who had vacated it without being able to sublet. PHCC bought the property and refurbished it to the practice's specifications. The total cost of the development was £1 250 000.

The District Valuer assessed the current market rent at £120 000. The health authority agreed to reimburse the rent and provide an additional sum allowed to the practice for taking on the responsibility for maintaining the building, through a full repairing and insuring lease. This means that the practice has much larger premises than would normally be reimbursed through the SFA assessment, at the price of taking on the risk of management and maintenance costs. The practice receives an additional 7% of the lease rental towards these costs, which the practice is currently investing. These lease negotiations were extremely complicated and time consuming and were handled by PHCC.

The only other costs incurred by the practice were legal costs and the installation of a new computer network. The physiotherapy room was equipped with money donated from a local charity.

Ownership and management

The building is owned by PHCC and leased to the practice under a 25-year lease. Responsibility for management of the facilities and the building has been taken on by the practice under the terms of the full repairing and insuring lease.

Service provision

The practice has four GPs, two of whom are part-time. There are two practice nurses, one of whom has particular responsibility for health promotion. The practice is a community fundholder and, through this, they employ a physiotherapist and purchase community nursing services. Counsellors, funded by the health authority and shared with other practices, run sessions from the centre. There is also a minor operations and treatment room.

Key features

This development would not have been affordable for the practice without the extra reimbursement from the health authority, in return for the practice taking on the responsibility for the upkeep of the building.

The expert knowledge that PHCC was able to bring to the financial and legal negotiations was seen as vital by both the health authority and the practice who lacked these skills in-house.

HEBDEN BRIDGE GROUP PRACTICE: WEST YORKSHIRE

Development:	Expanded GP premises
Funding:	Private developer
Timescale:	1995–January 1998

Profile

This project is a PFI to develop a new site for a GP practice currently based in a health centre. It involves the conversion of a disused mill, funded by a developer, to be leased to the practice with reimbursement through the rent reimbursement scheme. The final development will be larger than the existing health centre and will house additional primary care services and other planned developments such as day case surgery and remote diagnosis facilities.

Aims and key players

The initiator for this project was the Hebden Bridge Group Practice although, as the scheme developed, Calderdale and Kirklees Health Authority has assumed a facilitating role becoming the main negotiator with the local trust and the developer. The original plan was for a centre incorporating both statutory and voluntary social and health care providers. However, this initial plan has been scaled down to fit the funding available and to ease the development process.

The practice, a first-wave fundholder, is currently housed in a health centre owned by Calderdale Healthcare Trust. The practice has a list size of 18 000 patients and comprises ten GPs. The practice is motivated to move to larger premises to cope with an expanding practice population and to offer a wider range of services such as increased minor and day surgery, outpatient clinics and other developments which are as yet unspecified. By moving to their own premises the practice hope to be able to realise the potential of fundholding from a position of increased autonomy from the local trust.

These objectives fit with the wider strategic plan of the health authority. This involves moving some services into the community and a major reorganization of local secondary care provision within the next four years, including the provision of a new hospital in Halifax.

Funding

The lead GP initially contacted the developer who already owned and was to develop the disused property. They then jointly approached the health authority for funding for a centre that would incorporate the practice along with statutory and voluntary social and health care providers.

This original idea has been considerably pared down, reflecting the funding available and the difficulty of gaining a working consensus among a number of different agencies. The resistance of the practice to take such a large financial risk for premises not covered by GMS reimbursement was also a factor in reducing the scope of the development.

The proposal was not a market-tested development and therefore the health authority required professional advice to ascertain whether the proposal would pass various VFM and probity tests. This was provided by a property advisor, employed by the health authority and paid for by regional health authority pump priming funding.

The developer will fund the cost of converting and fitting out the building, with a guarantee of revenue from the 25-year lease with the practice and rent from a smaller area of commercial space in the building.

The health authority is currently negotiating with the practice over which additional services (over and above GMS) will be provided within the fundholding practice. This is expected to amount to approximately £75 000 worth of services per annum. The GP fundholding practice is expected to contribute a sum towards the ongoing costs of the building and this will be negotiated on the likely turnover activity. The practice will recoup maintenance money from contracts with the health authority. The health authority see the direct purchasing of non-GMS services from a GP practice as a move towards being able to specify quality and outcome criteria for these services.

At this stage, there has been an informal agreement with the trust that activity provided by the Hebden Bridge Group Practice will be costed at 15% lower than similar services provided by the trust. This 15% has been calculated as a rough estimate of the cost of capital to the trust. This means that, in order for the practice to break even on these services, they will have to be provided at a more efficient rate than currently operated by the trust.

The trust will have a reduced income to support their health centre when the practice leaves. In addition, the trust will lose part of their income that the health authority will use to fund the additional services provided at the practice. The trust will be unable to remove some costs from the system immediately as they are tied up in the overhead costs of running a hospital. The health authority and trust are currently negotiating this issue. However, it is the health authority's intention to reduce contracts by at least the variable costs and provide bridging costs until the new hospital allows further rationalization and enables the trust to reduce their costs.

Ownership and management

Ownership of the building will remain with the developer who will be responsible for facilities management for the 25-year period of the lease. The practice will pay a per-footage service charge.

Service provision

The following new service developments are confirmed for the new health centre with many other proposals at the development stage:

- a range of outpatient clinics including ophthalmology, gynaecology, paediatrics and mental health

- diagnostic facilities, including ultrasound and remote diagnosis along with chiropody, dentistry and physiotherapy services
- a minor and day case surgery suite including recovery areas is also planned.

It is envisaged that the facilities will become available for use by other GPs in the area once the health centre has been operational for some time.

The practice and the health authority are taking a pragmatic approach to service planning and they plan to see how the proposed service developments work before they embark on further developments.

Key features

The narrowing down of the initial plans to a GP-focused development enabled a shared vision to develop between the partners that might not have been possible, certainly within the current timescale, had many more providers been involved in the planning process.

The health authority sees its role in the PFI process as one of facilitation in order to make the proposals fit the GMS and HCHS funding available to support the development. In this case PFI has opened up new opportunities to work with developers and different designs rather than standard NHS solutions.

This development has required a high level of involvement by health authority staff in brokering the agreements and working out all the financial elements. Regional health authority pump priming funds covered some of these costs that would not be available for future developments. However, these costs should reduce over time as the health authority gains expertise in PFI developments.

HOVE POLYCLINIC: EAST SUSSEX

Development:	New premises for community and secondary health care services
Funding:	Trust and regional health authority
Capital cost:	£4 900 000
Timescale:	1991–1998

Profile

This development seeks to integrate community services and outpatient services provided by different trusts under one roof. It is consistent with the health authority's strategy for rationalizing services and was the result of a wide consultation and bidding process. The community trust is funding the majority of the development and will own the resulting building, with the acute trust as the main leaseholder.

Aims and key players

The origins of this development go back to 1991 and the formulation of the health authority's strategy to rationalize services involving the closure of Hove General Hospital. Separate proposals were submitted by both South Downs Health Trust (SDHT), a community trust, and Brighton Health Care Trust (BHCT), an acute trust and a local GP practice seeking to expand its premises and range of services.

Following a process of consultation involving GPs, the Community Health Council, Hove Borough Council, the trusts, local groups and residents, the SDHT proposal emerged as the preferred option.

Funding

The regional health authority provided £1.5 million, with the remaining £3.4 million raised by SDHT through land and property sales and leasing arrangements. The bulk of these property sales and expected service cost savings have arisen from the proposed relocation of mental health and community services on to the new site.

Ownership and management

The polyclinic will be owned by SDHT, with BHCT as the main leaseholders, and other organizations and practitioners charged on a sessional basis. The centre manager is employed by SDHT with plans to provide a joint reception service between the two trusts.

Service provision

The facilities of the polyclinic will be split approximately equally between the two trusts. Consulting rooms, diagnostic and therapy units, administrative areas and meeting rooms are planned. BHCT services will include a range of outpatient clinics and physiotherapy, radiology, x-ray and ultrasound and a pharmacy. There are plans to open a minor surgery unit in the future.

SDHT plan to base district nursing, health visiting, speech and language therapy, occupational therapy, psychology, chiropody and child health services at the polyclinic.

GPs will not be based in the polyclinic. Hove has many GP surgeries and it was not felt to be appropriate to place any one of them in the centre. The consultation with GPs at the beginning of the development process indicated that local GPs themselves were against GPs being sited in a polyclinic. However, there have been discussions about housing the local GPs' out-of-hours service at the polyclinic.

Key features

Housing services from two trusts in a building owned by one of the trusts has caused complexities throughout the development process. SDHT cite the amount of time devoted to developing a good joint working partnership with the main service providers, the funders and local community, as a prime factor in ensuring the success of the project.

The process of planning services to provide an integrated service for patients required the involvement of service managers at an early stage and emphasized good communication throughout the process.

KIVETON PARK HEALTH CENTRE: SOUTH YORKSHIRE

Development:	New premises for GP, community and voluntary services
Funding:	GP commercial loan and Rural Development Area (RDA) grant
Capital cost:	£1 025 000
Timescale:	1994–January 1997

Profile

Kiveton Park Health Centre covers a largely rural area which has been hard hit by the decline of the mining and steel industries.

There are high rates of both unemployment and preventable disease. The GP practice and the health authority worked with the Rural Development Area to secure funding for new premises housing the practice, community health services and voluntary organizations.

Aims and key players

The idea for the new primary care centre emerged from a good working relationship between the practice (a total purchasing pilot site) and the health authority. The doctors were looking to move from their cramped premises and had investigated a number of sites and cost rent options.

The health authority's strategy is to support the development of new primary care resources which meet local needs. The practice manager began meetings with the health authority, forming a good working relationship before any specific idea for development.

South Rotherham RDA, an agency of the Department of the Environment, had prioritised Kiveton Park as an area of particular deprivation and appointed a project officer to establish a local consultation forum. This body was responsible for submitting a successful funding proposal to the Department of Environment.

The practice employed a firm of architects to design a building that would meet the specifications collated from discussions with the local community, the health authority and local trusts.

Funding

The total capital cost of the development amounted to £1 025 000. The development has been primarily financed by a 30-year commercial loan taken on by the practice, with an RDA grant of £100 000 and fundholder savings contributing to the capital costs. Approximately half of the loan servicing costs will be met through the notional rent reimbursement scheme. Rental income from the community trust and other users of the premises will provide the remaining portion of the loan costs. The latter half has been underwritten by the health authority.

Ownership and management

The building is owned and managed by the practice who purchase community and acute services under standard and total fundholding arrangements.

Service provision

The centre houses five GPs. Community trust services include district nursing, health visiting and chiropody. Physiotherapy, community midwifery, minor surgery, occupational therapy and community psychiatric nursing services are also provided. As the centre is in a rural area, local people also use it for less serious casualty services. Voluntary groups can also use the building's facilities, e.g. the local Relate group operate a service from the centre.

Future plans for the centre involve the provision of pharmacy, dentistry and optician services. There is also a recognized need to overcome the initial hostility to the development from some GPs in the district.

Key features

Good partnership relations are seen as the key to the successful completion of this project. This has required a champion in both the health authority and the practice.

NEPTUNE HEALTH PARK: TIPTON

Development:	New premises for an integrated health and voluntary service centre
Funding:	NHS Executive regional office and City Challenge
Capital cost:	£3.2 million
Timescale:	1992–June 1998

Profile

A partnership development to provide GP, community health, secondary care and local voluntary sector services. Funding has been provided from the NHS Executive regional office via Sandwell Health Care Trust (SHCT) and a City Challenge grant via a local community association. The partnership formed to manage the development has worked hard to ensure commitment of all partners to the guiding principle of the social model of health.

Aims and key players

The development brings together four main partners, all of whom were working towards some form of integrated service provision. The health authority was responsible for pulling the schemes together.

- The *Black Country Family Practice* was looking for larger premises with the possibility of bringing in other services.
- Following a successful City Challenge bid, *Murray Hall*, a community organization that aims to support voluntary

sector and community development in Tipton, was granted £500 000.

- *Sandwell Health Authority* was looking to support local health services and had undertaken a local needs assessment that had shown a need for improved access to services.
- *SHCT*, a combined trust, was aiming to relocate community and outpost secondary health services in Tipton.

Funding

The development will cost £3.2 million. The cost of acquiring and reclaiming the site, £1.5 million, has already been met by the trust and City Challenge. An additional £500 000 from City Challenge will be routed through Murray Hall to finance their involvement in the project. The remaining capital will be provided by the NHS Executive regional office, via SHCT; the latter require an annual 10% return from purchaser contracts and lease rental on the property. The health authority will fund the GP element through the notional rent reimbursement scheme.

Ownership and management

The trust will own the building with leases held by the key partners. Although final management arrangements have yet to be agreed, the trust does not want to hold the day-to-day management responsibilities and it seems likely that a joint-funded centre manager will be appointed.

Service provision

A range of services has been planned including day surgery, endoscopy, minor injuries unit, x-ray, physiotherapy, audiology, chiropody, GP and community health services, a health bureau

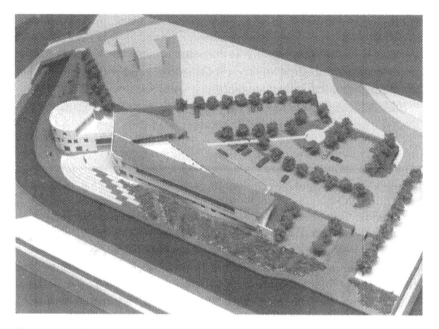

Figure 3.1: Neptune Health Park: model.

(run by Murray Hall), refreshment area, information centre, meeting rooms, a police base and crèche. Community nurses based in the centre will be largely linked to the GP practice. A minor surgery unit and a GP out-of-hours service will work in partnership with other GPs in the area.

There are discussions about letting space to private pharmacists, dentists and opticians and basing speech and language therapy services and a small ambulance unit on site. In the spirit of the principles that have led the development of Neptune, the trust is keen to ensure that the centre provides integrated nurse and practice-led services which meet local needs, rather than simply relocating hospital clinics. It wants to develop packages of care delivered jointly by service providers. Use of the physical space is to be kept as flexible as possible, with new ideas to be considered as they emerge.

Key features

The equal partnership approach and underlying commitment to the social model of health taken during this development, have allowed the resulting plans to be responsive to community needs. The process of reconciling different working cultures and beliefs has required a great deal of communication and commitment at all levels of the agencies involved.

NORTHWICH CENTRE FOR INTEGRATED CARE: CHESHIRE

Development:	New premises for community and secondary health care services
Funding:	Regional health authority
Capital cost:	£1.2 million
Timescale:	1995–July 1997

Profile

This involves the conversion of disused hospital accommodation and a new building to provide primary and some secondary care services, advice and information about local services and facilities for local voluntary agencies. The project involved capital costs of £1.2 million funded by the former North West Regional Health Authority, with some recurrent funding from South Cheshire Health Authority and joint funding for the centre co-ordinator by Mid Cheshire Hospital Trust (MCHT) and Cheshire Community Healthcare Trust (CCHT).

Aims and key players

The initial impetus for the development came from the health authority which was keen to encourage developments within the strategic context of shifting services towards a primary care-led NHS. MCHT, a predominately acute trust, had already expanded some secondary care services on the Victoria Infirmary site at Northwich.

The main aims of the development were to improve local access to a wider range of primary and secondary health care services and to integrate this provision with other statutory and voluntary agencies.

Northwich Health Forum was formed in 1995 to assess local health and social needs and to test the feasibility of establishing an integrated care centre in the locality. This forum has been the vehicle for joint planning of the project, under the chair of the chief executive of MCHT. Membership of the forum includes representatives from MCHT, CCHT, NHS Executive regional office, South Cheshire Health Authority, Northwich LMC (two local GPs) and Vale Royal Social Services. Figure 3.2 outlines the planning and consultation process undertaken by the Northwich Health Forum.

Funding

Following an option appraisal and community consultation process a bid was submitted to the regional health authority. This initial bid totalled £1.63 million, and was later reduced by removing elements such as the planned information technology links to GPs and the refurbishment of the administration area. This brought the bid within the £1.2 million available through a capital grant from the regional health authority. Due to the element of risk involved in renovating a listed building, a large contingency fund had to be set aside to fund unforeseen building costs. This fund

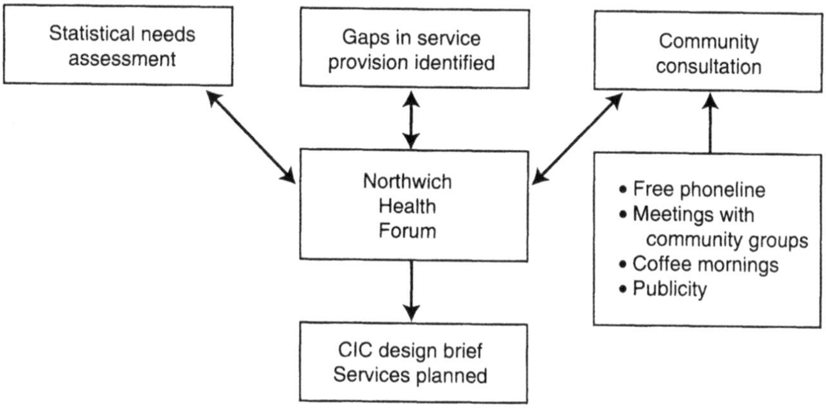

Statistical needs assessment	Gaps in service provision identified	Community consultation

| | Northwich Health Forum | • Free phoneline
• Meetings with community groups
• Coffee mornings
• Publicity |

| | CIC design brief Services planned | |

Figure 3.2: Centre for Integrated Care: planning process.

has since been totally absorbed into the building costs, although the project is not expected to exceed the original capital costs.

Ownership and management

The buildings will be owned by MCHT with CCHT as the main leaseholder. Day to day management will be provided by a centre co-ordinator, funded jointly by both trusts.

Service provision

Services will be a combination of new and relocated services including a full range of outpatient services and a telemedicine link to the district general hospital at Leighton. Day case surgery will be extended. Community health services, run by CCHT, will be based at the centre. Some integrated services will utilize skills from both trusts, including a 'hospital-at-home' scheme, respite and re-habilitation services, which will use the GP ward, and community nursing services. Training and teaching will also be key features for the new centre.

Accommodation for voluntary and community groups was a major part of the initial vision for the centre. The aim is for the voluntary provision to be linked with the appropriate clinics wherever possible. For example, the Centre for Visual Impairment will have a session booked to coincide with the ophthalmic clinic, and Age Concern will provide advice and information during the general medical clinics for the elderly.

Statutory support services plan to use the centre on a sessional basis at regular times. These include Benefits Agency staff and local authority housing advice workers.

Key features

Joint planning was seen as essential to the success of the project. Regular meetings and communication with staff about developments were important in ensuring trust staff support.

Local GPs have not been involved as much as initially anticipated and there is currently some concern within the trust that GP practices may be more interested in developing their own in-practice facilities and services rather than referring to, or using, the facilities at the centre.

RICHFORD GATE PRIMARY CARE CENTRE: WEST LONDON

Development:	New premises for GP practice, community trust services and commercial letting units
Funding:	London Initiative Zone (LIZ)
Capital cost:	£1 million
Timescale:	1993–June 1996

Profile

The Richford Gate Primary Care Centre is run by the Grove Medical Practice, a non-fundholding practice. The practice operates in West London with high unemployment and social deprivation. The practice had outgrown its premises and was keen to develop an integrated primary care centre with the local community trust. A local housing association agreed to rent part of an office block it was converting into flats to the practice to develop. The health authority allocated LIZ funding to the project that enabled it to be undertaken.

Aims and key players

The practice had been desperately seeking to move out of their previous building for ten years. A number of options were considered, including cost rent schemes, but they had all fallen through. During this time, the practice had developed a good working relationship with the health authority.

When LIZ funding became available the practice approached the health authority who agreed to use LIZ money to fund the capital development of the site. The health authority appointed West London Health Estates, an independent health development agency, to act on its behalf during the development process.

The aim from the beginning was to develop an integrated primary care centre with the local community trust, Riverside Community Healthcare Trust (RCHT). The trust was aware that there were inadequate community services in the area and a local centre to base services from was needed, but they had no capital to purchase such premises.

Funding

The capital cost of this development, approximately £1 million, came from LIZ money via the health authority.

The health authority made a substantial payment to Kensington Housing Trust (KHT) as a capital contribution towards the cost of rent over the 35-year lease period. The KHT were also paid a sum by the health authority to cover the accumulating interest charges incurred by them in purchasing the building before the finalization of lease agreements with the health authority.

The practice is able to pay the lease through a combination of rent reimbursement and rental income from RCHT and the commercial units.

Ownership and management

The health authority took on the lease for the initial two-year development period. On completion of the work, the GP practice took on a 35-year lease with KHT who remain the owners of the building. These complex legal and financial negotiations were handled by West London Health Estates (WLHE), the agency employed by the health authority to oversee the development process.

The practice is responsible for the building and service provision. The practice purchases maintenance services from RCHT to benefit from economies of scale.

Service provision

Services available in the centre include six GPs and two practice nurses, health visiting, district nursing, foot health, dietetics, palliative care, child psychology, physiotherapy, counselling, social work student placements, a seminar room facility, osteopathy and massage.

Apart from GP services, all services are run by the RCHT except social work and massage (both through an arrangement with Westminster College) and osteopathy (private practitioner). The Citizens Advice Bureau runs a weekly session from the centre. The building also houses three commercial units to be let to an optician, dentist and pharmacist.

Key features

Developments such as Richford Gate take a great amount of time and this can cause internal difficulties for participating agencies. In this case, it was the availability of LIZ money which made it possible to go ahead with such a large development. LIZ funding was seen as a source of flexibility and power that enabled a more ambitious and unusual development to be undertaken.

SHADWELL MEDICAL CENTRE: LEEDS

Development:	New GP-owned premises
Funding:	GP commercial loan
Capital cost:	£299 500
Timescale:	1993–November 1994

Profile

This practice took a gamble by purchasing premises that were too large to allow complete reimbursement under the SFA regulations. The result is a newly converted GP premises with two shop fronts and additional office space for rent. Funding was via a commercial loan taken on by the GP partners with revenue generated through notional rent reimbursement, rental from office and consulting space and two shops that financed the interest and capital repayments. It has allowed the fundholding practice to provide a wider range of services on site, increase its list size and take on a fifth partner.

Aims and key players

The development was entirely driven by the practice and their desire to move from cramped premises to cope with an expanding list size. The FHSA was originally approached by the practice for cost rent funding. Although sympathetic, the FHSA had no available funding for the development.

The development team comprised: a leading GP from the practice; an architect working for a small firm with experience of health service work; and a solicitor specializing in commercial property. The close working relationship they developed, together with their shared vision of the expected output, was seen by the practice as vital to the project's success. The District Valuer's expert advice was sought to determine the funding options available.

Funding

The practice reacted swiftly when a prime site, comprising 1.5 acres of land and an 8500 ft² building close to the main Leeds ring road, became available. Following discussions with an architect, the health authority and the District Valuer, the practice sought a commercial loan to cover the purchase and conversion cost of the premises.

Each partner contributed to a £4500 development fund that was used to pay professional fees. This fund enabled site plans to be commissioned, planning permission to be applied for and also gave a sense of commitment to the project from the other practice partners. The total cost (just under £300 000) was low for a development of this size because the premises could be converted rather than demolished and rebuilt.

The District Valuer advised on the regulations surrounding rent reimbursement. This allowed the architect to design the conversion based on the future notional rents and the requirements, as calculated by the FHSA, for a five-GP practice with space for a registrar.

The four partners who took on the loan established a separate property-owning partnership and VAT registered it. This enabled them to charge VAT on the rents and to claim back the VAT payable on building and development costs. This option is no longer available, since legislative changes to VAT mean that practices following a similar route now would incur 17.5% higher building costs.

The advantages for the practice undertaking the capital procurement and development process themselves meant they could proceed very rapidly and always felt in control of the development.

The projected reimbursement income was not sufficient to cover the additional running and loan financing costs of the new health centre. Therefore two shop fronts were developed; one with prior lease agreement from a local pharmacist, the other has since been let to an optician. Additional office space at the rear of the building has been let to Leeds Community Mental Health Trust (LCMHT) as a base for their community psychiatric nursing service.

Ownership and management

The building is owned by the practice with space leased to the various tenants on five-year full repairing and insuring leases. These leases give the tenants the right to vacate the property immediately if the practice leaves. An agreement with the pharmacist prohibits the practice from opening a pharmacy in the future and the lease with LCMHT prohibits the opening of a dedicated addictions unit on the property due to worries about drug addicts coming into the community.

Service provision

The move has enabled the practice to develop new services including minor surgery that may in the future be offered to other practices on a cost-per-case basis. Additional child health surveillance clinics, asthma clinics, diabetic clinics and health promotion clinics have been developed and physiotherapy and chiropody services are now offered by community trust staff on site. Close working relationships with the pharmacist and the community psychiatric nursing service on site have developed, with the practice benefiting from expert advice and quick referrals.

Key features

The speed at which this development progressed was unusual. Initial discussions were held in October 1993, building work began in April 1994 and the centre opened at the end of November 1994.

The comparatively narrow focus of the development, with a few, highly committed, key players and the fairly straightforward funding arrangements allowed the development to proceed at this speed.

The development fund was seen by the practice as important to the success of the project. It allowed the lead partner to make decisions rapidly and brought commitment to the development from the other partners.

The practice recognizes that the option to take on such a large financial risk is not available or attractive to all practices. The potential problems of negative equity, or being unable to gain adequate rental income, was not a major risk in an affluent area with an increasing population.

St Matthew's Health and Community Centre: Leicester

Development:	Converted premises for a multi-agency centre
Funding:	Regional health authority, health authority, NHS trust, charities and City Challenge
Capital cost:	£2 122 790
Timescale:	1994–August 1996

Profile

The centre is located in St Matthew's, an inner city estate with 4500 residents, which is one of the most financially and socially deprived communities in Leicester. Under the direction of a GP, the key players were brought together and funding was secured from a number of sources including City Challenge, NHS and charitable funds. Figure 3.3 gives an overview of the project.

The project involved the conversion of a large disused residential home on the estate and the relocation of a GP practice, community health services, and various statutory and voluntary services to the new premises.

Aims and key players

An ongoing problem for health and social service providers in the area has been the high rate of staff turnover and lack of opportunities for joint working. A partner at St Matthew's Medical Centre took the initial lead, encouraged by the results of a community needs assessment.

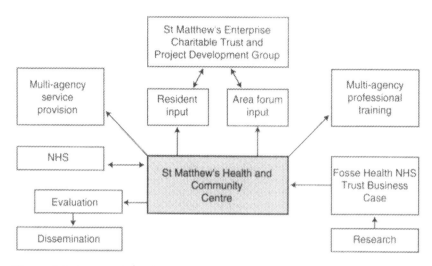

Figure 3.3: An overview of the St Matthew's project
(adapted from *Summary of St Matthew's Project*, February 1997).

A forum was established early on in the planning process to bring together the key players. These included the practice, Fosse Community Health Trust (FCHT), local residents and community groups, Leicester City Council and Leicestershire Health Authority.

Funding

The lead GP's petitioning raised the profile of the estate, the vision for the centre and brought many organizations on board. Following the first public meeting, local residents raised £1000 for the project. Substantial charity grants, totalling £249 700, were followed by capital funding of £150 000 each from the health authority and regional health authority. Savings from the relocation of trust staff and closure of other trust premises allowed the trust to contribute £1.2 million to the capital costs and to fund trust services at the new centre. The site of the centre, a former residential home, was sold to the project by Leicester City Council at a reduced cost. The council also provided funding for the centre's car park. The GP practice's rent is reimbursed by the health authority.

Ownership and management

The building is owned by FCHT, with the GP practice as the major leaseholder. Other services rent space on a sessional basis. Community groups can use the facilities free of charge. FCHT manage the building in conjunction with a project development group that decides overall policy and practice for the centre. The project is itself a charitable trust that can raise and distribute money for centre and community developments.

Service provision

FCHT operates district nursing, health visiting, speech and language therapy, community dentistry and community chiropody services from the centre along with administration work.

The GP practice is based in the centre. Other services include: the Leicester Mediation Service; a drugs and alcohol service; a domestic violence project; welfare rights; a legal advice service; the local police; the Benefits Agency; and a private optician's practice. The local mental health trust operates services from the centre and the social services department use rooms in the centre. Leicester University Medical School has a training unit based at the centre.

The centre also houses a meeting space, coffee bar, children's play area and community rooms available for local groups and trust staff.

Key features

While the development was a lengthy process, participants felt that this time enabled them to build a strong basis for joint working that has helped make the centre what it is. The involvement of local people was essential in producing a centre that meets their needs.

The role of the initiating GP was an important one in this development and helped to bring the key players and sources of funding together.

WEST END HEALTH RESOURCE CENTRE: NEWCASTLE

Development:	New premises housing a GP practice and health resource centre
Funding:	Regional health authority, City Challenge and Newcastle University
Capital cost:	£1.23 million
Timescale:	1989–May 1996

Profile

West End Health Resource Centre is a new building housing the University of Newcastle's General Practice Teaching Practice, and a Health Resource Centre (HRC) that provides community health services, leisure and fitness facilities, advice and information and facilities for community and voluntary groups. Developed by a private company, as part of a regeneration scheme for the local shopping centre, the capital costs of the centre were funded through a combination of regional health authority capital funding, a City Challenge award and a university grant. The Centre is a limited company and is administered as a charitable trust.

Aims and key players

The University Teaching Practice at Adelaide Medical Centre was the initial driving force behind the development, with the lead role taken by an individual GP. In 1988, the local authority put forward outline plans for the redevelopment of the half-empty shopping precinct in which the practice was situated at the time. The practice saw the opportunity to be involved in the redevelopment and to gain extra space and facilities.

The practice is situated in an area of Newcastle with particularly high levels of unemployment, households lacking car ownership, lone parent households and children in no income households. This economic and social deprivation is reflected in the generally poor health profile of the area.

The practice's initial objective was for a large health centre modelled on primary care resource centres to be a focus for all primary care professionals working in the locality. However, following a comprehensive needs assessment and consultation process with the local community (funded by a grant from the regional health authority), the proposals encompassed both social and health services.

In 1991, a steering group was established and comprised of representatives from Newcastle City Council, local GPs, social services, voluntary agencies, the local community and mental health NHS trusts, the FHSA, the regional health authority and local community groups. The steering group was responsible for running the project from this stage until the centre was opened.

Funding

The initial preferred option was costed at £1.75 million. Following bids, matched funding of £500 000 was pledged by the regional health authority and City Challenge. The initial proposal was re-assessed and downgraded to achieve a revised costing of £1 230 000. The University agreed to a £25 000 capital contribution and the regional health authority provided the remaining £205 000. Revenue consists of notional rent reimbursement to the practice, income from the leisure facilities and the leasing of consulting space, and charity and NHS trust funding for specific employment costs.

Ownership and management

The developer owns the building which is leased to the Centre on a 125-year lease with an additional service charge payable for maintenance. If the company becomes bankrupt, there is provision in the lease for the building to revert to the health authority and local authority. The practice sub-leases their premises from the centre with reimbursement through the notional rent scheme.

Overall management responsibility rests with the charitable trust established to administer the Centre. Membership comprises the city council, the health authority, the University, a GP and community representatives.

Service provision

Figure 3.4 outlines the main services provided at the West End Health Resource Centre. In addition to the full range of GMS provided by the GP practice, the following services have been developed at the centre:

- community information and advice

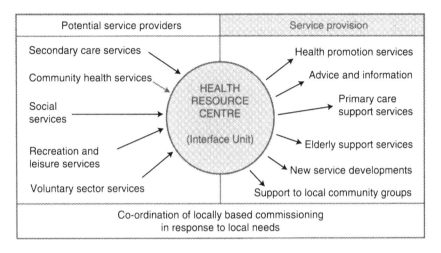

Figure 3.4: The West End Health Resource Centre concept (adapted from *West End Health Resource Centre Annual Report 1995–96*).

- a range of health promotion services provided in specific sessions by trust health promotion staff
- chiropody, physiotherapy and speech therapy services are provided by Newcastle City Health Trust through a licence agreement with the centre
- many health initiatives have been developed based on the gym and fitness facilities, e.g. a healthy workforce project for local NHS staff funded by local NHS providers
- a community health worker is employed by the centre, through joint funding with the community trust, to involve local people in developing local services.

Key features

The community needs assessment exercise, undertaken as part of the feasibility study, changed the direction of the project and may be responsible for its current acceptance and high usage by the local community. The approach taken by the project team, aimed at developing genuine local ownership, was time consuming and required close working relationships between all the partners involved.

4

Discussion and conclusions

It is the future of health services, to provide primary care and social care in one resource centre at the heart of the local community. (Kiveton Park)

GOALS AND OBJECTIVES

Despite their many differences, the innovative developments described in this book illustrate a number of common themes. The majority originated in the sometimes desperate need by a GP practice to find larger or better quality premises in order to take on additional partners to cope with an expanding patient list, to try and halt a declining patient list, or simply to improve the services that could be offered to patients.

A second common theme was the aim of developing and consolidating co-ordinated relationships between GP care, other primary and community health services and, commonly, local authority and voluntary sector services as well. Moreover, in the West End, Neptune, Kiveton Park and St Matthew's developments, concern about the overall inadequacy of local services and poor quality of life meant that improvements in the range and integration of local primary and community health were only part of a much wider range of social and economic measures to reduce local deprivation. The aim of widening the range of services available to the local community was also integral to the original impetus behind the Northwich Centre for Integrated Care; here, problems of urban deprivation were replaced by difficulties of access and poor transport to hospital services in a semi-rural area. Only one site, the Hove Polyclinic, originated from plans for a major strategic relocation of hospital services to the community.

Although severe pressures on general practice accommodation provided the initial starting point for many of these innovative capital developments, this did not remain the sole factor shaping their subsequent development. It is significant how many of the developments were characterized by opportunism and synergy. Thus an initial search for larger or better quality GP premises proved the starting point for a number of other organizations to join together and address a much wider range of objectives through a single capital development scheme. The most common additional aim was the rationalization and integration of primary care and community health services on a single site. Moving hospital services into primary care settings and nearer to local communities also became an objective that could be facilitated by primary care capital developments.

> We wanted a bigger building to be able to provide a lot more services and to be able to work with the community trust and put people in the primary health care team under one roof, because in the old building we could only have the health visitors in one cramped office, whereas here we can have the whole team. (Richford Gate)

Perhaps the clearest example of this synergy is the Neptune Health Park. A GP practice needed new accommodation so it could offer a wider range of services; the local NHS trust wanted to relocate community and some secondary health services; and the local community development organization was committed to tackling deprivation through increasing community involvement and participation in service planning and provision. All of these objectives in turn meshed with the health authority's service development and investment strategies.

> ... *One of the critical elements about the way we've worked is about putting partnerships together at the right time ... Our experience is that you end up with something you didn't invent. Nobody invented Neptune Health Park; we worked together and out of that collaboration came Neptune Health Park.*

In short, innovative and imaginative primary care development is not a straightforward, linear process in which service objectives are identified, capital secured and new premises constructed. The number of different professional and organizational 'stakeholders' who are likely to be involved in providing primary and community health services, and the variety of different capital procurement and revenue funding options together make it a much more complex process. The initiatives described in Chapter 3 illustrate the complex interactions between the priorities and objectives of different professional and community stakeholders, capital procurement opportunities and restrictions and pressures to secure long-term revenue income, within an overall regulatory framework that ensures public probity and value for money. Thus initial plans for service development could be modified by financial considerations (e.g. the need to secure a reliable source of revenue income might mean that community trust services, a pharmacy or an optician are incorporated into new GP premises); conversely, as service development strategies progress, changes may be needed in funding assumptions and building designs. Service development and capital developments in primary care are not separate, parallel processes but are complex and constantly interacting.

NEW SERVICE CONFIGURATIONS

The outcome of these complex development processes was a wide range of service configurations.

- Community health services, such as district nursing, community psychiatric nursing, speech and occupational therapy, community midwifery, physiotherapy and chiropody services. New premises enabled these services to be accommodated alongside a range of services provided by GP practice teams, such as clinics for patients with diabetes and asthma, child health and health promotion.
- Former hospital-based services, including minor and day surgery facilities, consultant outpatient clinics, diagnostic facilities such as x-ray and ultrasound and telemedicine links with district general hospitals.
- Non-health services that can nevertheless influence overall well-being and quality of life, such as welfare rights and legal advice, counselling services run by Relate and Family Mediation and support groups for older people, carers and young families. Many of the developments (St Matthew's, Neptune Health Park, Hove Polyclinic, Kiveton, Northwich and the West End Health Resource Centre) also provided meeting rooms for local organizations.

On the whole, other primary care services provided by pharmacists, opticians and dentists tended not to be part of integrated service 'packages'. Where they were located on the same site, this was more often because the financial balance sheet for the new development required a steady source of rental income that these tenants could provide.

Developments such as Hove and Hebden Bridge, which included a substantial number of former hospital-based services, were explicitly integrated into broader health authority strategies of moving services from hospitals to local community settings. The active support of purchasers is clearly essential if disinvestment in hospital-based services is to occur and contracts are to move to community settings.

FINANCIAL 'PACKAGES' TO FACILITATE CAPITAL DEVELOPMENTS IN PRIMARY CARE

The developments described in this book were deliberately selected to include a diverse range of capital procurement strategies. Three issues deserve particular attention.

1   Complex 'packages' of capital funding were often required, including funding from local and regional health authorities, NHS trust capital borrowing and revenue from land sales, private sector finance, central government regeneration funding and charitable donations. Sometimes various sources of capital funding were explicitly matched against each other. In the St Matthew's development, grants from the local and regional health authorities were matched and even the local people raised a small amount of capital, despite the community's high level of deprivation. Matched capital funding from the former regional health authority and City Challenge was also secured for the Newcastle West End Health Resource Centre.

2   'Packages' of capital for investment in new premises had to be accompanied by parallel 'packages' of revenue funding to provide secure sources of income and guarantee appropriate returns on that investment. Rental income from licenses or subcontracts to community trusts, pharmacies, opticians and other services were essential to the long-term financial viability of many projects, regardless of whether a GP practice, NHS trust or private developer was leading the capital procurement and development process. As part of putting together revenue 'packages', the District Valuer played a key role in advising on

the amount that would be reimbursed by the health authority to a GP practice under SFA regulations.

3 'Pump priming' finance could be very important in the early stages of a development, enabling feasibility studies to be carried out, land sites prepared and legal and professional advice purchased. 'Pump priming' money came from sources as diverse as charities (St Matthew's), GP practice partners (Shadwell), City Challenge (Neptune Health Park) and former regional health authorities (Hebden Bridge and Newcastle West End), though this last source is unlikely to be available in future. In Richford Gate, LIZ money provided flexibility and enabled the health authority to lease the property while the building conversion took place. Less tangibly, a relatively small amount of initial capital funding demonstrated a willingness to invest in a project or area, and this in itself could attract further sources of investment. For example, the development fund established by the Shadwell practice partners helped to cement their commitment to a development that carried considerable financial risks; the charity funding for St Matthew's was an impetus to attracting further funds.

It was actually charity money that set the ball rolling for funding ... money attracts money ... It adds a lot more than just us saying 'This is what we need here'. (St Matthew's)

THE 'PROS' AND 'CONS' OF DIFFERENT CAPITAL FUNDING STRATEGIES

Diverse local circumstances and constraints mean that no single capital funding strategy stands out above others. In reality, options may be limited and the advantages and disadvantages of particular capital procurement strategies need to be weighed against each other. What conclusions can be drawn from the experiences of these ten developments? It should be noted that although NHS trusts were involved in many of these developments, in only a few (Hove Polyclinic, Northwich Centre for Integrated Care and St Matthew's) did they play a leading role in procuring capital funding and leading the service planning process. The potential contribution of trusts to major new primary care initiatives is therefore not fully reflected in the following discussion.

SFA options and constraints

For any development involving GPs, the first source of potential funding is reimbursement through the cost rent and notional rent schemes set out in the statement of fees and allowances. These cover some of the revenue costs of supporting GPs' capital investment and certain running costs of the accommodation. A number of the projects reported that their initial plans had had to be considerably scaled down in size and/or scope, because the full costs of the proposed accommodation would not be covered by SFA regulations. Many of these constraints arose from the fact that the definition of GMS is widely acknowledged not to have kept pace with the increasingly diverse range of medical services that can now be provided in primary settings.

> *... the modern design principles around health care are that all the services will be on a single floor, that we get away from all the institutionalized images of health care, that we design in flexibility. (Kiveton Park)*

Forthcoming changes to these regulations promise to bring them more up-to-date.[1] However, problems may still remain with more community-oriented primary care developments that aim to involve local people and voluntary organizations in a range of non-clinical activities. Additional sources of capital funding (and associated revenue income) may still need to be found in order to build flexible, non-dedicated space for use by local organizations and community groups in inner city premises, with all the associated maintenance, insurance and security costs. In Kiveton Park, for example, a Rural Development Commission grant helped to cover these additional costs.

Nevertheless, even in projects like the West End Health Resource Centre, which aims to provide a focus for a wide range of community activities, it was acknowledged that the constraints imposed by current SFA regulations did make the GMS-related part of the building more compact and this, in turn, helped to keep down both capital and running costs.

GP-led initiatives

One of the developments, Shadwell, was managed throughout by the GP practice. The GP practice in the Belmont development worked in close collaboration with a private company specializing in primary care property development. For Richford Gate, an agency employed by the health authority provided professional and technical expertise to the project, working alongside the GP practice and community trust. Kiveton Park was also managed by the GP practice with support from the health authority. What factors contributed to the success of these GP-led schemes?

First, it was important to secure the commitment of all the partners in the practice. The Shadwell project was 'pump primed' by a development fund to which all the GPs contributed from their own assets and this helped to cement commitment to a scheme that carried considerable financial risk for the practice. Second, the GPs involved in these schemes commented on the high degree of control that they had been able to exert over the design of the new premises.

We weren't forced into anything we didn't want ... we're very choosy, we were very sure of the sort of building we wanted, the style we wanted and the quality we wanted. (Belmont)

... what an extraordinary difference it appears to make ... if the doctors are running it. We have a number of other buildings that are owned by trusts and ... trying to persuade trusts that GPs have legitimate interests! ... This [development] has broken a whole negative chain that has held back developments in health centres quite a bit. (Richford Gate)

Third, active GP involvement could enable developments to be completed relatively quickly.

The reason we did [proceed quickly] was that we bypassed all the admin, we didn't go for any improvement grants so we weren't bogged down by having visits from administrators or filling out forms galore, we just didn't bother with it. (Shadwell)

Fourth, because these practices owned or were the head lease-holders of their new premises, they could also control those parts of the building that were sublet to other services and could thus exercise some strategic leverage over the range of primary care services at a local level. (Of course, this leverage could also be used to resist potential competition or prevent the location of controversial services like drug and alcohol abuse services in an area, regardless of how much they were needed.)

The area has got a much better health centre with better flexibility, better pharmaceutical services, an optician and a base for the CPNs, and a dentist who has an expanded practice [based] in our old premises. (Shadwell)

On the other hand, GP-led schemes expose practices to considerable financial risks, including that of negative equity. For example, in Hebden Bridge, initial plans had to be scaled down because the GP practice was not willing to take on responsibility for securing funding for parts of the building that would not be covered by GMS-related reimbursement or health authority contracts. In addition, schemes involving GP practices as lead players created a considerable amount of extra work.

However, such risks and burdens could be considerably reduced. In the case of the Belmont Medical Centre, both financial risk and workload were almost entirely transferred to a private developer specializing in the primary health sector. This company bought the building, financed the conversion and negotiated planning permission with the local authority and the financial reimbursement package with the District Valuer.

> ... *the doctors had nothing to lose. We were the ones who took the financial risk. (Belmont)*

Health authorities could also help considerably in reducing the financial risk to GPs and providing assistance with particularly specialized aspects of financial planning. In the Richford Gate development, the health authority took a short-term lease on the new premises while the conversion took place and used LIZ money to underwrite some of the costs incurred by the housing association that carried out the development.

> *[LIZ money enabled] the health authority to get in there ... [and] be the tenant while the works were being carried out and then hand it all over to the GPs. It would not have been possible for the GPs to do it. (Richford Gate)*

A third strategy for reducing risks was for GP practices to share them with an NHS trust. In the case of St Matthew's the community trust funded most of the building conversion, while in Richford Gate the rental income paid by the community trust to the GP practice also reduced the practice's exposure to financial risk.

> *There is no way in an inner city area that any GP is going to buy a property under the cost rent scheme because of the difficulties. (St Matthew's)*

In addition to the risks and extra workload, GP-led developments and those where private developers work in partnership with GPs both tie practices to long (typically 25-year) leases or loan repayments. This is a considerable drawback when other changes in the primary care workforce are creating pressures for greater career flexibility and occupational mobility.

Private sector involvement

One of the developments, Belmont, was led by a GP practice in close collaboration with a specialist property investment and development firm. The PFI scheme at Hebden Bridge also involves close collaboration between a GP practice and a private property development company.

The value of private sector specialist expertise was undeniable. In Hove, the community trust employed a consultant who put together a Project Execution Plan to guide the different stages of the development process. A consultant was also employed to put together the full business case for the Neptune Health Park.

The negotiation for the lease was very important, you need a jolly good solicitor, preferably someone who is experienced in negotiating this sort of lease ... At the end of the day, it has been far less stressful than if we had done it ourselves, even if we had done a cost rent [scheme] ... because someone else has been doing the day-to-day running of it ... The third party approach, with something like the organization we have got here, means you are getting a lot of that expertise as part of the overall package. (Belmont)

The growth of property development companies specializing in smaller, primary care developments is clearly of considerable benefit to both GPs and health authorities, as they are likely to become highly knowledgeable about both the local property market and the various funding options offered by SFA regulations.

The work that is involved in putting together these projects with health authorities and doctors is much more than you have in any normal development project. The large developers are making a few noises but they really are not interested because the rewards are not there and it is too difficult for small developers. (Belmont)

However, expertise of this kind could have drawbacks. First, private developers, architects and contractors need experience of working with NHS clients, particularly in primary care settings. Failure to understand how the building would eventually operate could lead to apparently minor changes having unintended adverse consequences as outline specifications are translated into detailed plans and eventually implemented during construction.

I think there are all sorts of things we would have done differently if we had had our own architect working for us. (West End)

Second, there may be tensions between the commercial interests of private developers seeking to maximize profitability and the responsibilities of health authorities to ensure probity and value for money. The health authority involved in the Hebden Bridge PFI development needed to spend considerable time explaining NHS procedures and regulations to the private developer and ensuring these were adhered to. This is a particular problem in relation to formal PFI schemes, where clear procedures and approvals regulations have to be followed, and especially so where health authorities still have little experience of applying this process to primary care developments. The staff time involved in such negotiations, together with the purchase of quantity surveying and costing expertise not available 'in-house', was estimated to have cost £50 000 in the case of Hebden Bridge.

Third, there is a risk that the commercial interests of private developers may skew the primary care development process. For example, despite the extra workloads they had carried, the architect and GPs in the Shadwell scheme thought they had achieved a more efficient design than if a private developer had been involved. Because the latter would have been concerned to maximize profit from land sales, there would have been no incentive to create flexible, multi-functional rooms and thus keep down running costs. The health authority is clearly crucial here, in ensuring probity and accountability in the use of public sector finance to repay leases on PFI schemes, and the District Valuer in relation to cost and notional rent reimbursement for GP premises.

> *... we have got to be absolutely clear and accountable for the use of public money and one needs to have a rigorous mechanism in place to reassure and demonstrate that one has value for money in the use of public funds. And to my mind the District Valuer is the critical one in all that ... We have a responsibility ... to ensure that we are getting the best value for money. (Belmont)*

Finally, it may be that private finance is simply not available for certain kinds of primary care developments – ironically, those that are particularly badly needed in areas with very high levels of deprivation and poor services, especially outside London where land and property prices are low.

> *Neptune would not have happened if we had had to rely on PFI. Private finance can't see the benefits of something like Neptune, particularly if it is happening in a deprived area. (Neptune)*

In such circumstances, the formal requirement to appraise a planned capital development for PFI viability may seem irrelevant.

Multiple funding packages

Complex service developments may need to put together funding 'packages' from a number of different sources. The main drawback to this strategy is the length of time it can take; the West End Health Resource Centre, for example, took eight years from initial outline redevelopment proposals to official opening. Sustaining active commitment and involvement over such a period can be very difficult, particularly in local communities with a history of disinvestment and neglect.

> *... we had to keep the local population involved all the time which was very hard work ... their expectations have been met, they are not disappointed, which is one of the problems with these sorts of project where you get a lot of hype and then it doesn't happen. (St Matthew's)*

On the other hand, the sheer length of time that it can take to put together complex funding packages provides opportunities for the key stakeholders to establish good and effective working relationships with each other and cement the commitment of the organizations that they represent. Achieving effective inter-agency and interprofessional working relationships could be an important objective in itself, as well as being an essential means to the ultimate goal of a new primary care development.

> *I don't think you can underestimate the processes that you have to go through ... what is really behind this is a feeling, the spirit of Neptune, which is about trying to create more than just a building. (Neptune)*

> *What you don't want is a building opening and all these little islands of services not talking to each other. (Hove)*

THE ROLE OF HEALTH AUTHORITIES IN PRIMARY CARE CAPITAL DEVELOPMENTS

Health authorities play a crucial role in promoting and facilitating capital developments in primary care, even though they may not be the original initiators of such developments. For example, the Kiveton Park initiative originated with the GP practice but quickly won active support from a health authority keen to pilot new developments in the area. Health authorities are particularly likely to take lead roles in primary care capital developments where these form part of a broader strategy of reconfiguring hospital services and moving specialist services into the community, as in the Northwich Centre for Integrated Care and the Hove Poly-clinic. In Hebden Bridge too the health authority became a key player in negotiating the PFI scheme, because the GPs' plans for a new health centre would help further its wider strategy of relo-cating as many secondary services as possible to local, community settings.

Even without overarching strategic aims such as these, other health authorities were also reported to have taken a positive and opportunistic attitude to primary care premises developments, supporting them whenever the chance arose. This support could take a number of different forms:

- leading or funding local needs assessments that then forms the basis of a business case and service specifications, as in the case of the Northwich Centre for Integrated Care
- underwriting 'pump priming' expenditure to cover initial devel-opment costs (Kiveton Park) and the costs of PFI negotiations (as the Hebden Bridge scheme showed, these are likely to be initially high)
- providing or buying in specialist advice and expertise, to which GPs may not have ready access, in quantity surveying, financial planning and market-testing of primary care capital procure-ment options

  ... the importance of having a very well worked out plan and legal and financial structure before anybody starts spending big money. To get that is itself expensive, because you have got to pay lawyers, advisors and your professional team. (Richford Gate)

- liaising with the District Valuer over the cost rent and notional rent reimbursement likely to be available for new premises

- ensuring that value for money is obtained by GPs who work in partnership with private developers.

Health authorities also have an important role to play in managing the consequences of primary care capital developments. The consolidation of primary and community health services in new premises, or the transfer of services from hospital to new primary care settings can have major implications for other provider organizations, other GP practices and acute and community NHS trusts. Careful negotiations and sensitive transfers of contracts are required in order to maintain the viability and ensure the continued support of these other organizations. This role was particularly marked in the Hebden Bridge development, where the health authority planned to move contracts worth £75 000 p.a. from the local combined trust to the GP practice once it moved to its new premises. The health authority promised bridging funding to the trust until it could further rationalize its services and reduce overheads and running costs.

Similar 'knock-on' problems may arise for GP practices that remain in health centres after community health services have been relocated into new primary care premises. It will be important to ensure that these GPs are helped to maintain the quality of the premises in which their practices remain.

Major new capital developments raise wider equity questions, particularly if health authorities experience difficulties in funding new cost rent projects from pressurized, cash-limited GMS allocations and LIZ funding in the London area comes to an end. For example, although the health authority was pleased with the outcome of the Richford Gate development, it recognized that future developments on a similar scale would not be possible. Some health authorities were concerned about possible future cash limits on notional rent reimbursement and the consequent risk of entering into expensive reimbursement agreements with one or two 'flagship' primary care developments.

Each time one of these developments happens, we are locked into it … given it was a large sum of recurring money and given the benefits to that practice and the building ... but where did that stand in the greater scheme of things, across the whole of our practice population? (Belmont)

On the other hand, too great a concern with the equity issues arising from major capital and service investments can appear over-rigid and restrictive to GPs, trusts and other organizations keen to innovate and take risks. The role of health authorities in sustaining this careful balance between supporting innovation and protecting broader health objectives and interests will become even more important with the introduction of primary care pilot sites following the *NHS (Primary Care) Act 1997.*

One way of resolving this tension is for health authorities to play an active role in extending the lessons and experiences of innovative primary care capital developments to other GPs in the area. This is particularly important because of the potential competition between practices and the consequent resentment if one practice is seen to be given an unfair advantage. The experience of supporting a major new capital development can therefore be used to benefit primary care services across the area as a whole.

What we are now trying to do is to have that strategic plan and say, 'These are our one or two key premises we want to develop over the next 12 months' ... We are trying to learn from the Belmont Road development, and that is a method we may well want to use because it is a way of cracking into those barriers ... What is of bigger concern are deprived areas with lots of single-handed GPs, many of whom have a hard time just struggling by in their grotty premises, let alone thinking about doing anything clever and exciting on top. The trick for us is going to be about how we get this sort of arrangement for them. (Belmont)

Finally, active financial and other support from a health authority, especially when this was linked to wider strategic objectives, could give a degree of leverage over local primary care services and bring general practice within the scope of broader managerial initiatives to improve the quantity and the quality of local health care. This was the case in Hebden Bridge, where health authority commitments to move contracts to the new health centre were essential to the overall financial 'package'. The health authority was considering requiring the use of specified protocols and guidelines by the practice as a condition of these new contracts.

All these things start tying primary care in ... it reduces this crazy notion of independent contractors ... [If] you need health authority money you have got to go into partnership. (Hebden Bridge)

CONDITIONS FOR SUCCESS

What were the key factors that helped these innovative capital developments achieve their objectives?

Commitment from key individuals

All the developments had originated in the vision and determination of a single individual or small group of people; projects were subsequently taken forward through the commitment of these 'product champions' who were able to represent the interests of the main organizations involved. They played a number of important roles:

*   acting as spokespeople for the project – ... *we needed a leader figure to push forward the funding ... the one thing I would emphasize as very important for this project was the amount of outreach work. (St Matthew's)*
*   co-ordinating activities at key stages in the development process – ... *a core group ... to say 'We are going to do it, we are going to make it work. (Kiveton Park)*

- bringing in other organizations and resources when required – *Individuals have contributed by using their networks ... we would not hesitate to pull people in and out as it developed. (Neptune)*

It may be difficult to achieve an appropriate balance between involving all the key stakeholders throughout the development process and maintaining a steering group that is small enough to work efficiently and take decisions quickly. However, the sustained commitment of a few key individuals and a sense of 'ownership' and involvement in the project among a much wider constituency of purchasers, service providers and users are all essential.

Developing good working relationships

Developing shared objectives and commitment based on good communication and sound working relationships among the key partners was essential. Even if good working relationships did not exist at the start of the development, there was unanimous agreement that the *process* of development and planning should not be rushed so that these relationships had time to develop. This was particularly important where two NHS trusts were working together to plan services for a new centre (e.g. Hove Polyclinic and Northwich Centre for Integrated Care), or where statutory and voluntary sector organizations were working together for the first time (e.g. West End Health Resource Centre, St Matthew's and Neptune Health Park).

It was very sensitive to start with because both trusts applied to run the polyclinic. What was quite important, I think, was that there was a bit of a lull before we actually had to get together, to do the joint planning. (Hove)

Since ... we were made into two trusts, there hasn't been the same level of service between the two; this was an opportunity to improve this. (Northwich)

Considerable effort could be needed to overcome the competition, fragmentation and inflexibility created by the structures of NHS and other services.

We ... the doctors ... our concepts had come from community care ... getting used to the fact that social workers are people you can actually work with, voluntary agencies do their job ... Bringing everybody together was our aim, so we were a bit taken aback that people might be defensive about working with us! (Neptune)

Developing good working relationships during the planning and development stages was important because these would lay the foundations for the running of integrated services within the new centre.

The success of this scheme has been the joint working before we came here, but more importantly, the aim is to run it as far as possible as a single unit and that is fundamental. I am horrified when I hear of new developments with separate kitchens and staff rooms and all that. (Richford Gate)

We are trying to create something that is about integrated working and joint working ... What we don't want is everyone moving in here and doing their own thing ... (Neptune)

Expertise

A wide range of skills and experience is needed at different stages of major service and premises developments such as these. These will probably include District Valuers, project management skills, and the financial and technical expertise of architects, private developers and property advisors. Experience of applying these skills in the health care sector in general, and an understanding of the culture of primary care in particular, are of critical importance. It may be desirable for health authorities to take an active role in identifying and building up these sources of expertise, either in partnership with private sector finance, design and construction companies specializing in primary care development or through in-house or agency arrangements.

Timescales

Primary care developments that involve several statutory and voluntary partners, which access multiple sources of capital funding or which seek to bring together unusual combinations of services, all take time. Rarely were planning and construction completed to the original timescale, even where the capital procurement process was relatively straightforward. Most of the projects therefore emphasized the importance of realism in constructing project timetables.

> *If there is one key lesson, it is however long you think it is going to take, add 50% ... Do not underestimate the amount of time people need to plan and to think through what they actually want. (Hove)*

> *It is like eating an elephant – it has got to be done bit by bit! (Hebden Bridge)*

Involving local communities

Finally, the extent to which local communities and service users were involved in these primary care developments varied. Projects initiated and led by GP practices tended to consult users less than those that had broader objectives and explicit inter-agency and interprofessional agendas. The Neptune project, for example, used the community development organization, which had been set up under the City Challenge scheme, to consult with and involve local people in planning the new Health Park. Particularly where new models of primary care services are being planned, it will be vitally important to involve local people and community organizations to ensure that services actually meet local needs.

We very deliberately made it high profile public relations. (West End)

It needs good practice, someone who is capable of the management and who is also out there, encouraging local population and service ownership. (Kiveton Park)

SUMMARY AND CONCLUSIONS

A number of key conclusions emerge from these innovative capital developments in primary care.

Aims and objectives

Although most of the developments originated in efforts by individual GP practices to find bigger and better premises, they generally involved many more organizations and service providers in order to increase the range of services available to local communities or practice populations. These services included:

- primary care services – GPs, pharmacies, opticians and dentists
- community health services
- former hospital-based services, such as diagnostic facilities, specialist outpatient clinics and rehabilitation services
- non-health services provided by local authority and voluntary organizations.

Funding packages

The developments often needed complex 'packages' of capital funding from multiple sources; sometimes grants from different bodies were explicitly matched against each other. 'Packages' of revenue income also had to be constructed to cover the total rent, lease or capital repayment charges. These 'packages' were usually made up from SFA-related payments to GPs and rental or licence income from other service providers who used the new premises.

Although the SFA encouraged designs that were economical, it imposed constraints on the types and size of premises for which GPs could claim reimbursement. Proposed changes to the SFA may ease some of these pressures, although alternative sources of capital and revenue finance will probably still be needed for multi-purpose, flexible accommodation for informal, community use.

At present, full PFI schemes may not be an attractive option for primary care capital developments because of the relatively high costs of managing the small premises typical of this sector. In contrast, some of the capital developments were led by GP practices who procured capital from private sources, including private development companies. These schemes gave GPs considerable control over the development and could also be completed quickly. However, they could involve GPs in considerable financial risk and tie the practice to long-term lease commitments that reduced the partners' occupational mobility. This financial risk could be reduced through active support from the health authority and/or close collaboration with a local NHS trust, both of which can help to maximize the benefits of public–private partnership in capital developments.

The services offered by some private sector capital procurement and property development companies could offer risk transfer from GPs. However, previous experience of working with primary care partners was important and careful attention to probity and value for money issues were also needed.

The role of health authorities

Health authorities have a vitally important role to play in assessing local service needs, in providing access to specialist expertise and in managing the equity consequences of major primary care capital developments.

Success factors

- Planning new capital developments in primary and community health care depends crucially on networking skills and building relationships between organizations and professionals. The processes by which new developments are planned, funded and built, including the extent to which local communities are involved, will lay down essential foundations for effective joint working once the new premises are open.
- The continuing commitment of a few key 'product champions' is necessary to ensure continuity and maintain momentum; these individuals also need to work closely with their constituent organizations to ensure wide ownership of the new development.
- Planning new premises and developing new services are not separate activities, but need to take place simultaneously in order to maximize capital and revenue income options.

REFERENCE

1 Department of Health (1996) *Primary Care: Delivering the Future*. Department of Health, London.

Appendix 1

List of key contacts

for each case study

Belmont Medical Centre	Pauline Collins Practice Manager Belmont Medical Centre 53–57 Uxbridge Middlesex UB8 1SD	(01895) 233211

Hebden Bridge
Group Practice
	Philip Sands
	Director of Corporate
	    Strategy and Commissioning
	Calderdale and Kirklees
	    Health Authority
	St Luke's House
	Blackmoorfoot Road
	Huddersfield HD4 5RH
		(01484) 466000

Hove Polyclinic	Val Robbard Business Manager South Downs Health NHS Trust Brighton General Hospital Elm Grove Brighton BN2 3EW	(01273) 696011

Kiveton Park Health Centre	Alan Prigmore Centre Manager Kiveton Park Health Centre Chapel Way Kiveton Park South Yorkshire S31 8RF	(01909) 510100
Neptune Health Park	Dawn Wickham Project Manager Neptune Health Park Queen's Road Health Centre Tipton West Midlands DY4 8PX	(0121) 520 1101
Northwich Centre for Integrated Care	Liz Helbrough Hospital Manager Victoria Infirmary Winnington Hill Northwich Cheshire CW8 1AW	(01606) 564000
Richford Gate Primary Care Centre	Renos Pittarides Practice Manager Richford Gate Primary Care Centre 49 Richford Gate Richford Street London W8 7HY	(0181) 846 7555/7557
Shadwell Medical Centre	Dr Roger Potts Shadwell Medical Centre 137 Shadwell Lane Leeds LS17 8AE	(0113) 293 9999

St Matthew's Health and Community Centre	Stan Clark Director of Estates Fosse Health NHS Trust Gypsy Lane Humberstone Leicester LE5 0TD	(0116) 246 0100
West End Health Resource Centre	Dr Chris Drinkwater Senior Lecturer in Primary Health Care Department of Primary Health Care The Medical School Framlington Place Newcastle-upon-Tyne NE2 4HH	(0191) 222 7892

Appendix 2

Service provision by provider for each case study

Site	GP services	Community trust services	Acute trust services	Voluntary agencies	Other	Future planned services
Belmont Medical Centre	GMS• Minor surgery*	District nursing• Health visiting• Mental health counselling* Physiotherapy•				Minor injuries unit*
Hebden Bridge Group Practice	GMS• Minor surgery*	Chiropody• Dentistry• Day surgery• Diagnostics (ultrasound and remote diagnosis)* Outpatient clinics (ophthalmology, gynaecology, paediatrics, mental health)• Physiotherapy•				
Hove Polyclinic		Child health services• Chiropody• District nursing• Health visiting• Occupational therapy• Psychology• Speech and language therapy•	Diagnostics (x-ray, ultrasound)* Outpatient clinics (cardiology, chest medicine, rheumatology, obstetrics and gynaecology, midwifery, dietetics, phlebotomy, pain)• Pharmacy• Physiotherapy• Radiology•		Community rooms* Cafe*	GP out-of-hours• Minor surgery*

Site	GP services	Community trust services	Acute trust services	Voluntary agencies	Other	Future planned services
Kiveton Park Health Centre	GMS• Minor surgery•	Chiropody• CPN service• District nursing• Health visiting• Midwifery• Occupational therapy• Physiotherapy•		Relate	Meeting room*	Private pharmacy Private dentist Private optician
Neptune Health Park	GMS• Minor surgery• Out-of-hours•	Audiology• Chiropody• Day case surgery• District nursing• Endoscopy• Health visiting• Minor injuries unit* Physiotherapy• x-ray•		Murray Hall (health and community advice)* Citizens Advice Bureau*	Cafe* Crèche* Police• Meeting room*	Private pharmacy Private dentistry Private optician Speech and language therapy• Ambulance unit*
Northwich Centre for Integrated Care	Out-of-hours Co-operative	Counselling service* Family planning• Hospital-at-home• Integrated rehabilitation service• Liaison nurse• Night nursing service• Pain clinic•	Day case surgery• Integrated diabetic service* Outpatient clinics• Oral surgery• Pre-operative assessment clinics• Minor injuries unit	Age Concern• Centre for Visual Impairment• Citizens Advice Bureau• Cruise• Disability and Access Group*	Benefits Agency* Local authority housing advice* Teaching facilities* Meeting rooms*	Complementary medicine* Extended minor surgery* IT links to GPs* Four-bed MacMillan unit for hospice care*

Site	GP services	Community trust services	Acute trust services	Voluntary agencies	Other	Future planned services
Northwich Centre for Integrated Care (*continued*)		Palliative care[•] Respite for young disabled and chronically sick*	Telemedicine links*	Drug and alcohol agencies[•] Eclipse[•] ME support group[•] Motor Neurone Disease Society[•] Red Cross* Stroke Club[•] WRVS		
Richford Gate Primary Care Centre	GMS[•] Minor surgery[•]	Child psychology[•] Counselling[•] Dietetics[•] District nursing[•] Foot health services[•] Health visiting[•] Palliative care* Speech therapy*	Physiotherapy[•]	Citizens Advice Bureau[•]	Private dentist Private optician Private osteopath Seminar room* Social work placements[•] Massage*	
Shadwell Medical Centre	GMS[•] Minor surgery[•]	Chiropody[•] Physiotherapy[•] CPN service[•]			Private optician Private pharmacy[•]	

Site	GP services	Community trust services	Acute trust services	Voluntary agencies	Other	Future planned services
St Matthew's Health and Community Centre	GMS•	Chiropody• Community dentistry• District nursing• Health visiting• Speech therapy• Parenting project (includes paediatric outpatient clinic)*		Domestic violence project Drugs and alcohol service* Home Start• Leicester Mediation Service* Legal advice• Welfare rights•	Benefits Agency• Children's play area* Coffee bar* Community rooms* Police• Private optician• Seminar room*	
West End Health Resource Centre	GMS•	Chiropody• Health promotion* Physiotherapy• Speech therapy• Integrated elderly care team* Cardiac rehabilitation* Community health worker*		Rights project* Community Participation in Health (CHC)* Drugs and alcohol support group*	Community room* Crèche* Fitness and leisure facilities* Police•	Complementary therapies* Family therapy*

• Relocated services

* New services

Index